MW00878493

Published by: Baby Settler, LLC
For additional information go to www.babysettler.com.

ISBN: 9798726574301

Baby Settler: It's Not Just About Sleep.

*Navigate Feeding.
Establish a Routine. Get sleep.*

HILLARY SADLER

To my husband Luke, the first baby settler. Your unconditional love and support through the years is the only reason this book came to be. Your willingness and support to let me pursue my passions and dreams, as well as your constant clarity of mind and objective perceptions are, without a doubt, the reason Baby Settler has been able to bring confidence and rest to so many overwhelmed, exhausted parents.

TABLE OF CONTENTS

Preface

If you're reading this book, I'm guessing you have questions about breastfeeding, establishing a routine, and getting more nighttime sleep. Maybe you're a soon-to-be parent for the first time, or a seasoned parent who's looking for a refresher on how to survive the newborn days. Whatever your circumstance, you've come to the right place. This book will guide you on your journey to having a happy, settled baby.

Before we get started, I'd like to tell you a little about myself. When I had my first child, I had little knowledge about babies, either from reading or experience. I remember wanting to soak up all the information out there related to newborns and babies—and sleep! I did a lot of Googling, but it turned out that Google wasn't really helpful. Every baby is different. My baby isn't going to be the same as my sister's or my friend's baby.

Let me be real with you. The newborn period can be *very* challenging. Yes, it's typically a very joyous time in life, but it can also be an isolating time for new parents—particularly moms—whether you're a new mom for the first time or the fourth time. You have this newborn baby, and you're constantly feeding and changing diapers *all day long*. And you're trying to function on very little sleep.

When I had my first baby, I was completely overwhelmed with the newborn days. I had unrealistic expectations for my newborn. I had read all the books and thought I was well prepared. But nobody told me what the newborn period was *really* like. And that's why I'm going to tell you the real deal about babies and breastfeeding. If you follow these guidelines, you'll have a routine, get extended nighttime sleep, and thrive—not just survive!

I want to share something personal with you. I remember after having my first baby, I looked at him and thought, "This kid is draining me. He's already draining me, and he's only 5 days old! All I do is feed him, change his diapers, and try to get him to go to sleep. Is the rest of my life going to be just a series of feedings and changing diapers?"

Maybe you're feeling this way too but haven't verbalized it to anyone. It was a really dark place for me, and I felt completely alone and isolated, even though I had a supportive husband and family. If you're feeling the way I was, reach out to your OB provider so they can share some helpful resources with you. I regret not getting the support I needed sooner. Those dark feelings robbed me of time with my baby, and I can never get it back.

Now, no one debates the benefits of breastfeeding, *but man,* it can be a challenge! I would know. I didn't have it easy with any of my 3 children. Let's face it, breastfeeding is natural, but it isn't always easy. And that's the truth. Of the mothers and babies I've helped along the way, I'd say less than 50 percent have had it easy. It seems like there's always a bump in the road. In this book I hope to educate you, share helpful tips, and give you confidence to trust your intuition and make the best decisions for you and your baby.

Let me tell you a story. I was 4 days postpartum, exhausted, sobbing at the drop of anything, and I knew my baby wasn't getting enough breastfeeding. My husband called the lactation consultant we'd seen at the hospital and she said, "Feed the baby as much as he wants to eat, even if it's 12 times a day. That's normal." I was completely overwhelmed by that answer. I burst into tears and really couldn't see past the day. I wanted to breastfeed my baby, but I didn't think I could do it. All I thought about was, "How the hell am I going to sleep?" I became obsessed with finding a plan to get more sleep. The lactation consultant wasn't trying to make me feel defeated, but she wasn't giving clear, helpful information that empowered me. I thought, "If I'm going to breastfeed, my baby has to have unrestricted access to my boob 24/7. *I can't do that.*" It wasn't me. I needed structure, I needed a routine, and I needed sleep. I didn't breastfeed my first baby very long.

Making the decision to breastfeed is personal. No one has the right to make you feel pressured into breastfeeding. And no one has the right to make you feel like you can't breastfeed either. It isn't all or nothing. Every mom's baby and breastfeeding relationship is different.

As you're going through this book, I don't want you to feel like you're reading a strict manual. That would be exhausting. Especially if you're postpartum and not getting much sleep. I want this book to guide you. I'm sharing what you need to know to help your baby feed well and sleep even better. *And I'm equipping you to do it.*

With a few facts and practical tips relating to breastfeeding, *The Settled Baby Method* will educate and empower you to make informed decisions about *your* breastfeeding journey. So if you don't know anything about babies or breastfeeding, and you feel overwhelmed, you're in the right place! And if this isn't your first rodeo, I think you'll learn some new tips and find helpful tools. You'll be more confident figuring out why your baby's crying, and establishing a routine to get your baby sleeping through the night.

Since becoming a nurse, I've helped a lot of moms in the hospital setting over the years. I can relate to them. I understand their fears and frustration. But there isn't time in the hospital to share enough information to really support them. And I've realized that much information is lacking for moms who are breastfeeding.

Maybe this information isn't new to you. Maybe you've heard it before, but this time it makes sense. I hope after reading this book you will embrace your new role and feel confident that you *can* do this!

Are you ready? Let's go ahead and dive in!

The Settled Baby Method: Feed, Wake, Sleep and Have a Settled Baby

Sarah walked into the classroom exhausted and anxious. As her lactation consultant at the hospital, I had come to know Sarah and baby Emmeline very well over the past 8 weeks. She had been attending our postpartum breastfeeding support group every Tuesday until last week. In the early days, she and Emmeline really struggled with breastfeeding. In fact, Emmeline didn't latch or feed at the breast until about 5 days after birth. She was born a few weeks early, which was most likely a contributing factor.

I remember how defeated Sarah had felt those first few days after birth. She wanted to breastfeed more than anything. Their feeding plan consisted of using a double electric breast pump, finger feeds, paced bottle-feedings. Emmeline was on her own timeline, uh needed the solid stimulation from the electric pump to help her milk to come in. Sarah shed lots of tears over breastfeeding during the first 2 weeks of Emmeline's life.

When they didn't come to support group last week, I figured it was because they were doing so well that Sarah was feeling confident. But almost as soon as she sat down, tears fell down her cheeks. Breastfeeding had been brutal for her and Emmeline during the first couple of weeks, but I was happy to hear that the last several weeks they were doing amazingly well! Emmeline was gaining about 6 ounces per week. Because she was transferring 3 to 4 ounces at the breast, Sarah stopped pumping after breastfeeding. So if things were so much better, why was she here, and why was she crying?

Sarah wiped her tears and started to explain. She didn't come to support group last week because she was worried that I wouldn't agree with the strict schedule she had put Emmeline on once she reached 6 weeks old. She was excited because after the first 2 days Emmeline was sleeping 8 to 10 hours at night. I knew how important sleep was to Sarah. As a healthcare professional, she needed to return to work once Emmeline reached 12 weeks. Sarah's explanation caught me off guard, as we hadn't even discussed schedules or routines during support group. The extent of our conservations had been about what a great sleeper Emmeline was from day one. She was taking several solid naps during the day and was starting to extend her nighttime sleep to 6 hours when she was about 5 weeks old. I often commented about how efficient and effective an eater Emmeline had become, and I encouraged Sarah to keep feeding her on cue during the day to help extend her nighttime sleep. Sarah had never asked me specifically about a schedule—our relationship in the hospital and support group had been centered around lactation support.

Sarah said, "I think I've blown it. I put Emmeline on a schedule, and now she doesn't nap well during the day. She can barely make it 4 hours during the night before she becomes frantic. I spent about a week trying to implement the strategies I had read about how to help babies extend their nighttime sleep, but none of those strategies are working. We are both miserable, and I'm more exhausted today than I've ever been. Finally, my husband said, 'Are you sure she's getting enough to eat?'

"It was like a slap in the face, realizing that I'd been letting a schedule and book dictate how and when I cared for my baby. The last few days I've paid attention to her feeding cues, and I've been feeding her when she wakes from a nap. If she seems hungry, I've allowed her to eat 30 minutes earlier than the schedule says. And the shift has happened. She's back to taking her solid daytime naps, and she's starting to extend her nighttime sleep again."

Sarah was so upset she could barely speak. She was trying to figure out a schedule that would be beneficial for her and Emmeline. She had worked so hard to establish a good breastfeeding relationship with her baby, and she wanted to continue to breastfeed. She also wanted to establish a routine and feel confident that she would have uninterrupted nighttime sleep as she transitioned back to work.

Sarah was disappointed in the number of available resources pertaining to routines or schedules for breastfeeding moms. Most of the books and online courses that aimed to help parents get their baby on a schedule and sleeping through the night were missing the most important pieces of the puzzle—education and support.

I'm all too familiar with Sarah's frustration. I was exhausted, strung out, and overwhelmed. I felt guilty that my baby was not exclusively getting breast milk. I couldn't figure out how to continue breastfeeding or pumping while getting my baby on a schedule so she could sleep through the night and I could get the rest I desperately needed.

So I developed a method that allowed me to enjoy a healthy, balanced life, knowing my baby was being well taken care of. My baby was now on a routine I could count on, and I was able to plan my day and get at least 8 hours of restorative, uninterrupted sleep every night. This method allows one-on-one time with my spouse, a break from being needed 24/7, the mental capacity to go to nursing school, to finish my master's degree, to become an International Board Certified Lactation Consultant, to create an online video course, and now, to write this book. What is the method? It's *The Settled Baby Method: Feed, Wake, Sleep and Have a Settled Baby.*

I'm Hillary, the founder of Baby Settler. I'm also a mom, a nurse, and a lactation consultant. I've spent my entire nursing career working with mamas and babies as a bedside nurse in labor and delivery and postpartum, a newborn transition nurse (catching babies), and a lactation consultant.

Over the years my patients would look me up on social media with questions about general newborn and infant care and feeding. They wanted to know how to soothe their newborn. They asked, "Why is my baby crying all the time?" "Is my baby getting enough to eat?" "Will I ever sleep again?" They had questions about breastfeeding and maternal mental health as it relates to breastfeeding. They were interested in both my personal and professional opinion—because Google wasn't giving them the information they needed. While there are many resources available, the excessive amount of information and, in many cases, the complex format often leave parents feeling even more confused. Parents need evidence-based facts and helpful tips and tools, written in a straightforward format, that encourage confidence in their ability to trust their intuition and decision-making capabilities.

Only *you* really know what is best for *your* unique child.

I've helped many parents who felt paralyzed and unable to make decisions about their life and specific circumstance because the books they read or courses they took didn't outline how to handle the X, Y, and Z that they were currently experiencing. Your baby just isn't going to fit into the template created by someone else.

While you're reading this book, imagine that I'm sitting in your home with you, having a friendly mom-to-mom conversation about key topics, pertinent tips, and suggestions from personal experience while helping you gain confidence through evidence-based information, not just my opinion.

The contents of this book will be your guide as you establish a routine that you can plan your day around and have a baby that sleeps "like a baby" at night. Whether breastfeeding or bottle-feeding, you will feel confident in your ability to figure out what your nonverbal baby needs to be a happy, content baby who sleeps through the night.

The Settled Baby Method: Feed, Wake, Sleep and Have a Settled Baby will help you navigate each stage of life, from birth through your baby's first year.

Feed

Learn how to get efficient,
effective feeds to get more sleep.

CHAPTER 1

Breastfeeding: Getting Started

When you first start breastfeeding, you're in the initiation stage. There are a few things you should be aware of during this initial stage. I don't want to get too technical here, but I want you to know how it works—how you make breast milk. It's important to understand because this information will help you troubleshoot and problem solve down the road. You will use this knowledge to help your baby sleep through the night.

MILK PRODUCTION

Breastfeeding is all about supply and demand. After you deliver your baby and placenta, you'll get a surge in hormones. The hormones involved with breast milk production are prolactin and oxytocin. Prolactin is responsible for *making* milk, and oxytocin is responsible for *moving* milk.[1] Oxytocin also helps your uterus contract after delivery. If you are concerned that you have an inadequate supply of milk, you might have retained placental fragments, which can affect your breast milk production.[2]

Here is an example: In a special care nursery, a new mom was pumping exclusively because her preterm baby wasn't ready to breastfeed. She was 2 weeks out from delivery and only able to pump 10 to 15 ml each time. She had been pumping 8 times a day as advised. This inexperienced mom was unsure of how much breast milk she should get when pumping and felt concerned that she should be producing more. So she made an appointment to see a lactation consultant. The consultant reviewed her history and agreed that something was going on. She asked the mother if she had noticed any cramping when she pumped. The mother said no. Since she had only been pumping on the minimal stimulation setting, they made a plan to increase the setting to see if it helped with production. Within 24 hours of increasing the suction, the mother had a delayed postpartum hemorrhage. She underwent a D&C to remove any retained placental fragments left in her uterus. Within a day she began to see an increase in her breast milk production, and it changed from yellow colostrum of the initial milk to transitional and then mature milky white that suggested her milk was fully "in."

Why am I telling you this story? I want you to know two things: First, retained placenta can affect milk production. If you ever feel that your breast milk is not transitioning, or not "coming in," the cause could be retained placental fragments. This condition is often

---

1 Westerfield, K. L., Koenig, K., & Oh, R. (2018). Breastfeeding: Common Questions and Answers. *American Family Physician*, 98(6), 368–373.

2 Huang, L., Xu, S., Chen, X., Li, Q., Lin, L., Zhang, Y., Gao, D., Wang, H., Hong, M., Yang, X., Hao, L., & Yang, N. (2020). Delayed Lactogenesis Is Associated with Suboptimal Breastfeeding Practices: A Prospective Cohort Study. *The Journal of Nutrition*, 150(4), 894–900. https://doi.org/10.1093/jn/nxz311.

overlooked. Secondly, the hormone oxytocin is a key component of breast milk production. If your baby is feeding vigorously at the breast, you're likely getting the surge in oxytocin that you need. But if you're pumping without adequate suction, or feeding a preterm baby, jaundiced, or a baby with a high percentage loss of birth weight who has a weak suck, it could adversely affect your breast milk supply.

FEEDING ON CUE

During the first 2 weeks of breastfeeding, it's important to *feed on cue.* I hesitate to suggest how often to feed during this time because moms interpret that as a scheduled feeding plan, which I don't recommend. But your baby *and your breasts* need feedings at least 8 times in each 24-hour period.[3] The feeds might be every 1 1/2 hours, every 2 hours, or every 3 1/2 hours.

Your baby will feed most efficiently and effectively when you're feeding on cue.[4] That means your baby will feed the fastest, get the fullest, and sleep the longest. It doesn't mean you'll be an open buffet for the remainder of the time you choose to breastfeed. I'm talking about *the first 2 weeks of life.* This information, right here, is what my lactation consultant didn't tell me. More on this in chapter 3.

Here's something else you should know. The hormone prolactin doesn't act like you might expect. It'll peak after about 20 minutes and then steadily decline, even if your baby is still breastfeeding after 45 minutes. Many women think the goal is to breastfeed for a longer duration so they can make it longer between feeds and get more sleep. Let me tell you why it doesn't work like that.

3 Chen, Y.-J., Yeh, T.-F., & Chen, C.-M. (2015). Effect of breast-feeding frequency on hyperbilirubinemia in breast-fed term neonate. Pediatrics International : *Official Journal of the Japan Pediatric Society, 57*(6), 1121–1125. https://doi.org/10.1111/ped.12667.

4 Watchmaker, B., Boyd, B., & Dugas, L. R. (2020). Newborn feeding recommendations and practices increase the risk of development of overweight and obesity. *BMC Pediatrics, 20*(1), 104. https://doi.org/10.1186/s12887-020-1982-9.

SUPPLY: NON-NUTRITIVE SUCKING VS. SUCK-SWALLOW RHYTHM

Your newborn baby will only feed vigorously for about 15 to 20 minutes at a time. Typically he'll feed on one side and fall asleep, then you'll burp him, wake him, and feed him on the other side for 10 to 15 minutes. In the first couple weeks of life, newborns aren't going to feed vigorously for more than about 20 to 30 minutes at each feeding. Your baby might be doing non-nutritive or comfort sucking but not transferring milk. *The time spent at the breast comfort sucking does not count as active feeding time.* It's really important that you know the difference between non-nutritive sucking and a suck-swallow rhythm. To the untrained eye, it can be hard to differentiate between the two. When your baby is doing non-nutritive sucking (NNS) or flutter sucking, he is not transferring breast milk. Therefore, he may be "feeding at the breast" but is not getting any breast milk volume. When babies transition to NNS at the end of breastfeeds, after going through the suck-swallow rhythm, this is normal. However, if your baby is only doing NNS, this can lead to dehydration. If you're not sure, ask your baby's provider to show you the difference.

Back to the hormone prolactin. Its job is to make milk. To have an increasing milk supply you need increased prolactin levels.[5] Remember how it peaks after about 20 minutes, then starts to drop even if your baby is still feeding? To increase your breast milk supply, it's better to feed your baby more frequently for shorter durations than to feed fewer times for a longer duration. Your body will get more spikes in prolactin levels when you do an extra feeding or two. And it's almost pointless to push your baby past his feeding time limit of about 20 to 30 minutes during the first few weeks of life. Feeding on cue—your

5 Golan, Y., & Assaraf, Y. G. (2020). Genetic and Physiological Factors Affecting Human Milk Production and Composition. *Nutrients, 12*(5), 1500. https://doi.org/10.3390/nu12051.

baby's cue—will result in more efficient, effective feeds, and therefore more sleep for you and your baby.

I took care of a patient who was readmitted to our special care nursery because the baby had low blood sugar, hyperbilirubinemia (jaundice), and 14 percent loss of birth weight. Born on her due date with no complications at delivery, she had been breastfeeding at least 8 times a day, according to her parents. As I assisted with a feeding at the breast, I immediately identified the problem. Her parents thought she was feeding well, but she was only engaged in non-nutritive sucking. *She wasn't actually transferring any breast milk.* All the problems that had developed were a direct result of her weak suck at the breast. The jaundice, weight loss, and low blood sugar prevented her from getting over the hump. Her weak comfort sucking hadn't been enough stimulation for her mother's milk to make the full transition from colostrum to transitional or mature breast milk. We developed a supplemental feeding plan for the baby and a breast pumping plan for the mother. She was discharged a few days later, fully feeding at the breast. I'm telling you this story because I want you to know how important it is to know the difference between active sucking and swallowing versus non-nutritive sucking.

FEEDING DIFFICULTIES

Let's talk about complications that can occur in the early days of breastfeeding. The first concern is weight loss.[6] It's normal for your baby to lose weight after birth. But when your baby is approaching a total loss of 8 to 10 percent of her birth weight, she might not breastfeed vigorously. This weak suck can lead to a delay in your milk transitioning and coming in. When there's a delay in mom's milk coming in, the baby does not gain back her birth weight. I see this

6 Tawia, S., & McGuire, L. (2014). Early weight loss and weight gain in healthy, full-term, exclusively-breastfed infants. *Breastfeeding Review, 22*(1), 31–42.

all the time. When babies have lost about 10 percent of their birth weight, I recommend that mom starts pumping after each feeding until her breast milk is transitioning and her baby's weight is on the rise again. This helps mom get more stimulation and spikes in prolactin and oxytocin, which results in greater breast milk production.

Also, if mom has any expressed breast milk from pumping, I encourage her to give it to her baby via a supplemental technique, which we will discuss. Most babies who have lost 10 percent of their birth weight begin to feed better at the breast when being supplemented with expressed breast milk or formula. This method is referred to as a triple feed. And it can be overwhelming and exhausting. It's important to have both a lactation consultant guide you and a supportive partner to help. I recommend having your partner feed your baby with the supplemental method while you're pumping. That way everyone is done at the same time and can rest until the next feeding. Babies who are jaundiced may also have feeding difficulties like this. They tend to be very sleepy, and their lazy feeds can affect mom's supply.

NIPPLE SHIELDS

Let's talk about nipple shields. I have a love-hate relationship with these things. I love them when used appropriately—they can really help a baby latch who wouldn't have been able to otherwise. But I hate when they're used unnecessarily and therefore cause unnecessary issues.[7]

While not always necessary, indications for using a nipple shield are: preterm baby, flat or inverted nipples, a high palate, mom's anatomy, baby's anatomy, and simply not being able to hold a latch. These are the most common reasons for using a nipple shield.

---

7 Coentro VS, Perrella SL, Lai CT, Rea A, Murray K, Geddes DT. Effect of nipple shield use on milk removal: a mechanistic study. BMC Pregnancy & Childbirth. 2020;20(1):N.PAG. https://doi:10.1186/ s12884-020-03191-5.

It's important to use the right size shield. There isn't a one-size-fits-all solution, and using a shield that isn't fitted correctly can cause trauma to your nipple or limit the amount of breast milk your baby is able to transfer at the breast. Ask a nurse or lactation consultant to help you with sizing.

There is a technique to putting the shield on as well. It doesn't just sit on top of your nipple. If you're using a shield, be sure you know what a good latch looks like. If your baby is just sucking on the tip of the shield and doesn't have the entire shield in his mouth, he won't get as much milk as he could. When using a nipple shield during the initiation stage of breastfeeding, I recommend that moms double pump after feedings. It helps to ensure you're getting adequate stimulation so there isn't a delay in your milk transitioning and coming in. Once your milk has come in, you don't need to pump anymore.

Most women become anxious about weaning their baby off the shield, and it's important that this doesn't become a major source of stress. Attempt to latch your baby without the shield a couple times each day. Don't spend more than a few minutes doing this. If your baby starts to get upset, put the shield on and try again later. You don't want your breast to become a place of stress for you or your baby. Keep it a happy place. You can always try latching without the shield after feeding. Your baby might be more inclined to attempt something new when he's not hangry.

PACED BOTTLE-FEEDING: FLOW RATE

Did you know you can give your baby a bottle *and* breastfeed? Let's talk about something I'm super passionate about: paced bottle-feeding. A lot of people have never heard of this. Paced bottle-feeding is a technique—a way to give your baby a bottle if you want to breastfeed and bottle-feed. When you hear the term "supplementing," it can be referring to supplementing with breast milk or formula. It's simply a term used for breastfed babies.

There are several techniques used to supplement babies with breastmilk or formula, including cup feeding, syringe feeding, finger feeding, supplemental nursing system, and bottle-feeding. Many parents are concerned about bottle-feeding and how it will affect breastfeeding. I've seen many preterm babies who had been primarily bottle-fed transition to breastfeeding almost exclusively once they were older and stronger. Although there might be slight nipple confusion, most often the problem with a baby no longer breastfeeding after taking a bottle is related to the *flow rate*.[8]

Here is a real-life example: A mother is breastfeeding her baby who is only 36 hours old. He's been breastfeeding well but is starting to cluster feed, and his mom is exhausted. He's feeding as frequently as every hour. Mom is concerned that he isn't getting enough at the breast. Her nurse and lactation consultant assure her that he's doing exactly what they expect him to do—cluster feed. It's perfectly normal, and there *is* an end in sight. They educate her on expected output and signs of dehydration, which could include a high-pitched cry, a sunken fontanel, dry mucous membranes, jaundice, excessive weight loss (over 10 percent loss of birth weight), lethargy, inability to wake for feedings, uric acid crystals in diaper, and decreased or no passing of stool. This list is not all-encompassing. They also show her how to hand express and remove colostrum, so she is confident that he is getting colostrum when he feeds. He continues to cluster feed, and she becomes anxious and asks for a bottle of formula. But she hasn't learned about paced bottle-feeding. She gives her baby 2 ounces of formula in less than 5 minutes and continues this throughout the night. The next day, she's upset because she can't get her baby to latch.

---

8   Zimmerman, E., & Thompson, K. (2015). Clarifying nipple confusion. *Journal of Perinatology, 35*(11), 895–899. https://doi.org/10.1038/jp.2015.83.

The lactation consultant explains that the flow rate of the formula out of the bottle is much faster than the flow rate of the colostrum out of her breasts.

In this case the latch issue was caused by the *flow rate* of the bottle-feeding, not the formula or the bottle. Paced bottle-feeding is imperative when you're breastfeeding and bottle-feeding. Your baby will get frustrated at the breast if he's getting a fast flow of milk from the bottle. Pacing your baby when giving a bottle will help him to be content with going back and forth between breastfeeding and bottle-feeding.

Scientific evidence suggests that the primary reason for babies being unable to go back and forth between breastfeeding and bottle-feeding has more to do with flow rate and less with nipple confusion.[9] With paced bottle-feeding, you're positioning the bottle so that your baby is only getting milk when he's actually sucking.

The next time you're ready to bottle-feed, try this: Tip the bottle upside down and you'll notice it drip, drip, drip. If you put a bit of pressure on the tip of the nipple, it will start flowing. Hold your baby in a laid-back position and prop the bottle in her mouth. If she has the slightest bit of suction on it (or maybe no suction at all), and it's just running down the back of her throat, she will keep swallowing because she is unable to control the flow rate. She will keep feeding even though she may be full, because her option is to either swallow or choke. Paced bottle-feeding helps promote infant-driven feeding.[10] Infant-driven feeding is beyond the scope of this book, but many studies prove that infant-driven feeding is beneficial to babies, whether breastfeeding or bottle-feeding.

9 Kotowski, J, Fowler, C, Hourigan, C, Orr, F. Bottle-feeding an infant feeding modality: An integrative literature review. *Matern Child Nutr.* 2020; 16:e12939. https://doi.org/10.1111/mcn.12939.

10 Spill, M. K., Callahan, E. H., Shapiro, M. J., Spahn, J. M., Wong, Y. P., Benjamin-Neelon, S. E., Birch, L., Black, M. M., Cook, J. T., Faith, M. S., Mennella, J. A., & Casavale, K. O. (2019). Caregiver feeding practices and child weight outcomes: a systematic review. *The American Journal of Clinical Nutrition,* 109(Suppl_7), 990S–1002S. https://doi.org/10.1093/ajcn/nqy276.

It's important to pay attention to your baby's feeding cues—feed her when she's hungry and stop when she's full.[11] Of course, this is good practice for anyone. When we're eating, isn't it recommended that we stop right at the point of fullness so we don't overeat? Keep that in mind when you're feeding your baby.

---

11 Hurley, K. M., Cross, M. B., & Hughes, S. O. (2011). A systematic review of responsive feeding and child obesity in high-income countries. *The Journal of Nutrition, 141*(3), 495–501. https://doi.org/10.3945/jn.110.130047.

CHAPTER 2

Breastfeeding: How Do I Know My Baby Is Getting Enough?

FREQUENCY AND DURATION

During the first 4 to 6 weeks of life, your baby can be expected to eat *at least 8 times* in 24 hours. In order to grow, your baby needs to eat many small amounts, due to the size of her stomach.

Whether breastfeeding or bottle-feeding, you need to understand the concept of frequency and duration. When we discuss the frequency of a feed, we're talking about the time interval between the first feeding and the next feeding. For example, if your baby feeds at 9 a.m. and then at 12 p.m., that is a 3-hour feeding interval. When we discuss the duration of a feed, we're referring how long it takes her to feed. So if you want your baby to eat within a 3-hour time interval, if she starts feeding at 9 a.m. and it takes her 30 minutes to feed, then you only have a 2½ hour break between feeds. Does that make sense? Again, the frequency refers to the time interval from the start of one feed to the start of the next feed, and the duration is how long it takes your baby to feed. So remember, from birth until 4 to 6 weeks, your baby needs to eat at least 8 times in 24 hours to take in the volume and calories she needs to grow.

Now, there are exceptions. You may think your baby can take 7 feeds and be fine. This may be true for a larger baby who is bottle-feeding and can take in more volume with each feed. But overall, my statement applies to the majority of newborn babies during the first 6 weeks of life.

The volume of breast milk or formula your baby needs at each feeding is based on the weight of your baby. If you're breastfeeding, you don't know exactly how much he's getting at each feeding, so how do you know he's getting enough?

When your baby is finishing a feeding, you'll notice him relax his clenched fists and transition to a non-nutritive suck. He will likely unlatch from the breast or bottle and have a period of alertness as well as content sleep between feeds. These are all signs that your baby is getting enough milk. During infancy, follow up regularly with your baby's provider to confirm that breastfeeding is going well.

Remember, at birth babies will lose a percentage of their birth weight. This is not concerning—it is normal. However, we don't want to see them lose more than 10 percent of their birth weight. They should stop losing weight by day 3 or 4, and gain from 4 to 7 ounces a week after those first couple days. By about 2 weeks old, babies should be back to their birth weight.[12]

12   Tawia, S., & McGuire, L. (2014). Early weight loss and weight gain in healthy, full-term, exclusively-breastfed infants. *Breastfeeding Review*, 22(1), 31–42.

SNACK FEEDING

To ensure good healthy feedings during your baby's fourth trimester, or first 12 weeks, it is important to avoid snack feeding. You want to help your baby organize her feeding throughout the day. What do I mean by this? If your baby gets into the habit of eating small volumes every hour around the clock, she won't get good quality pockets of sleep. This turns into a vicious cycle of eating a little and falling asleep, then waking after 30 minutes because she is truly hungry due to just a snack feed an hour ago. She feeds again but not vigorously, and she is not getting a full feeding because she's tired. She falls asleep too soon and wakes up hungry within an hour. And the cycle continues. Does this sound familiar?

Let me clarify. More frequent feeds *are* better for mom's supply. However, I'm referring to *full feedings* every 2 to 3 hours, not a "snack" feed every 30 to 45 minutes. The actual time spent at the breast can't necessarily be your threshold or gauge point. Some babies will empty a breast (take a full feeding) in 5 to 10 minutes, and other babies will spend almost 30 to 40 minutes at the breast to get a full feeding.

SUPPLY AND DEMAND

Here is something I really want you to hear. This piece of the puzzle often gets lost with mothers who are breastfeeding, and much of the sleep difficulty experienced during infancy can be traced back to this: *For breastfeeding babies, the amount of breast milk your baby takes in at each feeding is different each time.* Your baby is not going to eat the same number of ounces at each feeding. Just as we feel hungrier at different times of the day, your baby does too. Your baby will stop breastfeeding when he is full. Your breast milk supply will change throughout the day as well. For example, you will have a greater supply during morning feeds than you will at 5 p.m. It's just how your body works. This doesn't mean you have a supply issue.

When a breastfed baby is feeding at *scheduled* times, it may prevent him from getting his daily caloric needs met. Now I'm not saying you can't have a routine to your day—in fact, I think you should, as you will see. What I'm saying is this: If your baby is hungry at 9:00, but you delay the feed because he's not scheduled to eat until 9:30, your body will think your baby wasn't hungry until 9:30 even though your breast milk was available for him at 9:00. If your baby is tired from being held off and as a result doesn't breastfeed very well, then your body thinks he really didn't need that much breast milk; it adjusts to that cycle and decreases your supply. This is the main reason why breastfeeding moms start to see a supply and demand issue with their baby. When a breastfeeding mom doesn't feed on cue, she risks her body's ability to be in tune with her baby's needs.[13]

ENGORGEMENT

Having engorged breasts is not equal to having a lot of milk. Some women are concerned that if they don't have engorged breasts, their baby isn't getting enough milk. This is a common misconception. Please understand, engorgement is *not* a good thing. When you have engorgement, you have breast tissue compression, which leads to breast milk suppression.

Here is a real-life example: A mother delivers her baby and is breastfeeding on cue from day one. The baby is now 3 days old and has jaundice. He's very sleepy with feeds and isn't nursing as vigorously as he had been. Mom's milk starts to transition, and her breasts feel painful and engorged. The baby is only feeding for 5 to 10 minutes at each feeding. Mom's breasts are not able to soften between feeds because her baby is not emptying them. Her breasts stay engorged

13 Davie, P., Chilcot, J., Jones, L., Bick, D., & Silverio, S. A. (2020). Indicators of 'good' feeding, breastfeeding latch, and feeding experiences among healthy women with healthy infants: A qualitative pathway analysis using Grounded Theory. *Women and Birth.* https://doi.org/10.1016/j.wombi.2020.08.004.

for 2 to 3 days. Now the baby is a week old. He's more alert, starting to feed better, and his bilirubin level has gone down. He has woken up and realizes he's hungry! The mother starts to worry because it seems like he isn't getting enough when breastfeeding. She reaches out to a lactation consultant, and it is confirmed that her breast milk volume isn't adequate for what her baby needs. The lactation consultant helps with a plan to get her breast milk supply in tune with the needs of her baby.

What happened here? The mother's breasts were engorged for several days and were not being emptied at each feeding. Her baby was not feeding vigorously, so her body thought it didn't need the breast milk. Also, the engorgement caused suppression of breast milk. The takeaway is this: While you might experience some engorgement when your milk is transitioning, you shouldn't have constantly engorged breasts.

Here are some things you can do: Take over-the-counter, non-steroidal anti-inflammatory medication, such as ibuprofen, to help with breast tissue inflammation. Use heat before feeding or pumping. Use cold for about 10 to 15 minutes after feeding to help with inflammation. Your breasts should feel a little fuller at the start of feeds, but it isn't ideal to have hard, engorged breasts before feeds. Engorgement is not proof that you have a good supply. After the initial transition from colostrum to mature milk, most women whose supply is in tune with their baby's needs do not have engorged breasts between feedings.[14]

BABY'S STOMACH

It is important to know the capacity of your baby's stomach. This will help you to be more confident during the period of time you're

---

14 Gresh, A., Robinson, K., Thornton, C. P., & Plesko, C. (2019). Caring for Women Experiencing Breast Engorgement: A Case Report. *Journal of Midwifery & Women's Health, 64*(6), 763–768. https://doi.org/10.1111/jmwh.13011.

waiting for your breast milk to fully come in. The initiation and colostrum stage of breastfeeding can be very challenging. As we've noted, many women worry that their baby isn't getting enough milk. It helps to know that during the first 24 hours of life, your baby's stomach is only about the size of a cherry! It holds about 5 to 7 ml at each feeding. That's only a teaspoon. By day 3 your baby's stomach is about the size of a walnut, and is able to hold just under an ounce at each feeding. By the end of the first week, your baby's stomach is about the size of an egg and can hold between $1\frac{1}{2}$ to 2 ounces at each feeding. After about 2 weeks, when your milk has fully transitioned, your baby is able to take anywhere from 2 to 4 ounces at each feeding during the first 4 to 6 weeks of life.

CLUSTER FEEDING

Are you feeling stressed and worn out? Your baby is probably cluster feeding. Cluster feeding means close-together feedings. There will be many times during your breastfeeding journey when your baby will cluster feed. It happens within the first 24 to 48 hours after birth. We talked earlier about supply and demand and how a woman's body makes breast milk. Cluster feeding is the way your baby tells your body she needs more milk.

So what is this like in real life? It is exhausting! Your baby may breastfeed for what seems like a full feeding, fall asleep for 10 minutes, then wake up again *acting hangry.* She might breastfeed for 5 minutes, stop feeding, act fussy and uncomfortable as if she isn't "getting anything" at the breast, have hiccups, feed again, fall asleep during the feeding, and then wake up ready to feed again! Does this sound familiar? You are not alone!

Cluster feeding occurs primarily during the first 6 weeks, but it can also happen during developmental leaps and growth spurts, as well as in the evenings. Evening cluster feeding can help your baby extend nighttime sleep by consuming more calories. If you look at the recommended routines at the back of this book, you'll notice that evening feeds are clustered together. *Clustered feedings are key to extending nighttime sleep.* If you try to "hold off" your baby from feeding during the early evening hours, it can work against your desire to extend nighttime sleep.

Here are some examples of how this works: If your baby hasn't had a poopy diaper in a few days, you might notice him being less interested in breastfeeding. Maybe his feeds are shorter in duration, or maybe he's dropped a feed or two for a few days. Your body will start to adjust to his new feeding pattern if he feeds this way for 2 to 3 days in a row. Then he'll have a blowout, his belly will feel better, and he'll be ready to eat like normal again. It takes a few days to get your supply back in tune with what he needs, so he'll do some cluster feeding to help send the message to your body that he's ready for more milk.

When breastfeeding babies are sick, and especially when you are sick, they may have a feeding pattern similar to the one I just mentioned. Your illness and their irregular and less vigorous feedings can affect your supply in the same way, and your baby will probably cluster feed during or after the illness.

Remember, at the end of the day your baby will get fewer ounces per feed than he does in the morning. *That's one of the main reasons breastfeeding babies cluster feed in the evenings.* So let him cluster feed! It will help to extend nighttime sleep. Other factors such as being overstimulated or overtired can also affect nighttime sleep, but don't ignore the feeding aspect of the equation when trying to troubleshoot nighttime sleep issues.

LET'S REVIEW

Breastfeeding babies should be back to their birth weight by 2 weeks old and gain about 4 to 7 ounces per week after the first 2 weeks. Keeping track of your baby's wet and poopy diapers will help ensure he's getting enough nourishment. By the end of the first week, he should have at least 6 wet diapers and 3 to 4 poopy diapers every 24 hours. Your baby should have periods of alertness after breastfeeding, followed by periods of content sleep. It's normal to have days where your baby cluster feeds, but if he is constantly acting hungry, you should reach out to a lactation consultant.

It's important to assess whether or not there is something concerning going on when your baby is having really long feeds and slow weight gain. You need to assess how much your baby is transferring at the breast. This won't be an exact amount, because she'll transfer more at some feeds than others based on how hungry she is at any given feed. But if you find that she only transfers 15 ml or a half ounce at the breast and she's 4 weeks old, this is a serious concern. A situation like this may mean there is a supply issue.[15]

Please note: If after the first 6 weeks your baby is needing to feed for at least 40 minutes at each feeding every day, has slow weight gain, and seems to need to eat 10 or more times each day, there could be a problem with the latch or with your milk supply.

LACTATION CONSULTANTS

I've helped many exhausted moms who were desperate to make breastfeeding work. They couldn't figure out why they were having issues and were exasperated.[16] Sometimes it's the latch. Sometimes it's mom's supply. It could be any number of reasons. You need to utilize a lactation consultant to help you figure out the best plan mov-

15 Kent, J. C., Ashton, E., Hardwick, C. M., Rea, A., Murray, K., & Geddes, D. T. (2021). Causes of perception of insufficient milk supply in Western Australian mothers. *Maternal & Child Nutrition, 17*(1), e13080. https://doi.org/10.1111/mcn.13080.

16 Coelho de Moraes, I., de Lima Sena, N., Ferreira de Oliveira, H. K., Saldanha Albuquerque, F. H., Carneiro Rolim, K. M., Verganista Martins Fernandes, H. I., & Chase da Silva, N. (2020). Mothers' perceptions of the importance of breastfeeding and difficulties encountered in the process of breastfeeding. *Revista de Enfermagem Referência, 2*, 1–6. https://doi.org/10.12707/RIV19065.

ing forward. And let me tell you, there isn't a one-size-fits-all lactation consultant! If you've had a bad experience, please try to work with someone else. I have met some LCs who have the unapproachable mentality that no matter what, "breast is best," and they ignore the real complications that can and do happen.

My work as a lactation consultant combines academic knowledge and practical training in specialty areas with personal experience, having had issues breastfeeding my own children. I help moms troubleshoot and make a plan that works best for them. So if you've had a bad experience with a lactation consultant, I am really sorry. And again, I urge you to find the one that you jive with!

RISKS FOR LOW BREAST MILK SUPPLY

Let's talk about reasons you might have a breast milk supply issue.[17] There are several medical conditions that can affect your supply. I will mention these conditions, but if you need further support, please reach out to a lactation consultant.

- Postpartum hemorrhage: One condition that can affect your supply is a severe postpartum hemorrhage. If your blood loss at delivery is over 1000 ml, I would recommend you start pumping as soon as possible. Breastfeed your baby on cue, and follow feedings with a breast pump session. Pumping will help your prolactin and oxytocin levels to spike more.

- Delayed transition: Be aware of the potential for a delayed transitioning of colostrum to mature milk, and make sure your baby isn't showing signs of dehydration while you're in the waiting.

- Magnesium sulfate: Another complication in delivery is related to magnesium sulfate. If you're getting an IV infusion of magnesium before labor due to high blood pressure or preterm labor, this can also affect the timing of your milk coming in. Ask your nurse to set you up with a breast pump immediately following delivery.

- Retained placenta: We discussed retained placenta frag-

17 Whitten, D. (2013). A precious opportunity: supporting women with concerns about their breast-milk supply. *Australian Journal of Herbal Medicine, 25*(3), 112–126.

ments earlier in this book. Remember, a retained placenta can affect milk supply.

- Breast deformity: Another high-risk factor for low supply is a history of a breast deformity or underdeveloped breast tissue. If you've had breast surgery, there is the potential that milk ducts were severed.

- Hypothyroidism: Untreated hypothyroidism can affect milk supply. I always tell moms who have a history of hypothyroidism to keep in mind that it can affect breast milk production if your thyroid levels are out of whack. If there is a concern, get your thyroid levels checked.

- Hormones: Polycystic ovarian syndrome can also affect supply.

- Other factors: Smoking, high blood pressure, anemia, and even diabetes can contribute to a low milk supply. Having any one of these conditions doesn't mean you won't be able to breastfeed, but they can potentially affect breast milk supply. It is important to work with a lactation consultant as needed.

Communication is vital. Have an open conversation with your baby's provider about breastfeeding, because sometimes things can get missed. It is crucial that you discuss your health history. Otherwise, if your baby is slow to gain weight or you are questioning whether or not he is getting enough at the breast, your provider might continue to promote exclusive breastfeeding when your baby really does need to be supplemented.

Pediatric providers are typically very supportive of parents who want to breastfeed because it is proven that breastfeeding has many benefits. I completely agree. But I have seen how withholding information can cause problems.

Consider this scenario: You have a history of a breast deformity and had breast surgery in your twenties. You go to the hospital and deliver your baby. Breastfeeding is going well and the latch is good. You've started this journey without a hitch. Now, 2 or 3 weeks later, you're completely exhausted and feel like there are signs that maybe your baby is not getting enough to eat, but your pediatrician says,

"This is normal; babies cluster feed, and breastfeeding babies feed anywhere from 8 to 12 times in 24 hours. So you think, "Okay, this is normal. This is normal. This is how it is." But in reality, because of your history of having a breast deformity, maybe there really *is* a supply issue. Perhaps your breast tissue isn't fully developed and able to make breast milk. It's possible that your baby really isn't getting enough at the breast. If your pediatrician had known about your history, it would have clued her in on the potential for a milk supply issue, and she would have considered that your baby really wasn't getting enough at the breast.

In this example, I'm not saying this mom can't breastfeed her baby, but she may also need to supplement after feeding at the breast. Her best solution is to reach out to her local lactation consultant for an in-person evaluation of the breastfeeding relationship to find out how much breast milk her baby transfers at the breast.

CHAPTER 3

Feeding on Cue from Day One

SIGNS OF HUNGER

Your baby will feed easier, require less stimulation to stay awake, and transfer more breast milk when you are feeding him on cue. This means you're looking for signs of hunger in your baby. What are these cues? Early feeding cues are when your baby brings his hands to his mouth, transitions from sleeping to waking, turns his head from side to side, sticks out his tongue, smacks his lips, clenches his hands into a fist, or becomes restless.

Crying is a late feeding cue. It's always more difficult to get your baby to latch when he's crying. Pro tip: If you're starting a feeding with a late feeding cue, place your baby against your body. The skin-to-skin contact will calm him down before latching. It also helps if you latch him onto your clean finger and let him suck for a few minutes prior to transferring him to latch to your breast.

THREE REAL-LIFE EXAMPLES

Here are some real-life examples of feeding on cue: The first couple had a newborn, only 2 days old. They had been struggling to get him to wake up for feeds. The baby was swaddled in the bassinet and going to town on a pacifier (we'll discuss pacifiers later). I offered to help with a feeding, but the couple declined and asked if I would come back in an hour, which was his scheduled time to feed. They were feeding him every 3 hours. I explained how the hormone prolactin works with breastfeeding and encouraged them to feed on cue rather than scheduling his feedings. They insisted that they would like to wait until his scheduled feeding time, so I agreed to come back later. After an hour, the couple called me to their room. The pediatrician had come in to see their baby and said that he was approaching a 10 percent loss of his birth weight. She was concerned and wanted to be sure the couple had a solid feeding plan for going home. We attempted to wake the baby for the feeding, since it had been about 3½ hours since his last feeding. He was frantic at first, disorganized, and difficult to latch. He finally latched and gave a few good sucks. However, he very quickly fell asleep at the breast. The couple explained that it had been a chore to get him to feed vigorously. He was eating for less than 10 minutes at each feeding. I pointed out the difference between non-nutritive sucking and active suck-swallowing. They agreed that most of his feeds had been non-nutritive sucking, and they really hadn't noticed him swallowing. Feeling very concerned about his weight loss, they asked me to help them figure out a plan so they could continue to breastfeed. Again I explained the importance of feeding on cue and assured them that it would result in their baby having more effective feeds. I also promised them that feeding on cue would help promote restful pockets of sleep. I encouraged the mom to pump after feedings until her milk came in, because her baby wasn't feeding very vigorously and was at a 10 percent loss of birth weight.

The next couple were second-time parents. Having struggled with breastfeeding with their first baby, they came into it this time with eyes wide open. They had made similar mistakes to the previous couple by insisting on scheduled feedings the first 2 weeks. The mother ended up with a breast milk supply issue and had to start supplementing with formula. This time their approach was different. I assisted with latching, and the baby was actively sucking and swallowing at the breast. After feeding, the mom was anxious to hook up to her breast pump in order to avoid having supply issues this time around. She had been pumping for 15 to 20 minutes after each feeding, and I assured her she was off to a great start. Her baby was feeding effectively at the breast. The mother was feeding on cue and getting adequate stimulation from her baby's suck for her breast milk supply to be in tune with what her baby needed. But we needed to have a conversation about another problem—overstimulation and the potential of creating an oversupply. This scenario has its own complications, which we'll discuss later. She thanked me for the information but was adamant that she wanted to pump after each feeding. A few weeks later she called, upset that her baby wasn't latching easily due to her forceful letdown and oversupply. She was constantly engorged and in pain. If she didn't pump every 2 hours, she'd end up engorged and unable to care for her children due to her painful breasts. She had clogged ducts, and it was only a matter of time before she developed mastitis. I wasn't surprised to hear from her. Her routine from the first day had caused her body to think she was feeding twins, when she only had one baby.

The last couple got it right. They were realistic with their expectations. They understood how breast milk production works and about potential complications that could come up. They had been feeding their baby on cue, about every 1½ to 3½ hours. They looked for early feeding cues, and that's when they started feeds. Their baby was feeding for about 15 to 25 minutes at each feeding. They weren't following a schedule, but they planned to follow a "feed, wake, sleep cycle" during the first few months of their baby's life. It had been working great so far. Their baby was ready to eat upon waking, and they noticed that if they missed feeding cues, or if they delayed feeds, it made the latch more difficult and their baby wouldn't feed vigorously. I encouraged them to continue to feed on cue. They were doing a great job! I asked if they were getting some rest, and they both said, "Yes!" They admitted that feeding on cue was more effective and required less stimulation to wake their baby. I followed up about a week later, and the baby was above birth weight, they were feeding about 8 to 9 times a day, and they were getting one 4-hour stretch of sleep at night. They felt confident that their baby was getting enough breast milk and had no concerns.

PACIFIERS

We can't talk about feeding on cue without talking about pacifiers! Is it okay to use pacifiers? How do I know if my baby is hungry or just wants to suck on the pacifier? The answer to these questions can be confusing, so I'll give you some solid guidelines and hopefully a little clarity.

The American Academy of Pediatrics recommends using a pacifier to promote safe sleep,[18] but the World Health Organization's 10 steps to successful breastfeeding says not to give any pacifiers or artificial nipples to breastfeeding infants. So, which is it?

I recommend waiting to introduce a pacifier until after breastfeed-

---

18 Task force on Sudden Infant Death Syndrome. (2016) SIDS and other sleep-related infant deaths: Updated 2016 recommendations for safe infant sleeping environment. *Pediatrics. 138* (5) DOI: https://doi.org/10.1542/peds.2016-2938.

ing is well established.[19] For most breastfeeding babies, that's usually after the first 2 weeks. After that time, mom's milk is usually in and baby is hopefully latching without any issues.

Why do I recommend waiting 2 weeks? Because if your baby is sucking on a pacifier when he's hungry, it can affect your milk supply. I've walked into many hospital rooms where parents have given their newborn a pacifier because they were trying to make it to the 3-hour scheduled feed. Now you can see why this is an issue!

To recap, if your baby isn't allowed to feed on cue or cluster feed, but is sucking vigorously on a pacifier instead, your body is not getting the message that your baby needs more milk. This can negatively affect your supply. When your baby is latching well, your milk has transitioned and come in, and you're committed to learning your baby's feeding cues, then using a pacifier isn't going to interfere with breastfeeding.[20] Just be sure you're not using the pacifier to hold your baby off for feedings, unless you're in a situation where it's absolutely necessary.

A good rule of thumb is this: If your baby sucks on the pacifier and falls asleep within a few minutes, he probably wasn't hungry—he just needed to suck to help soothe. If he's sucking vigorously on the pacifier and is irritable and alert, he's probably hungry. Feed him.

These three stories represent real-life scenarios. Hopefully they will illustrate how important it is to feed on cue.

19 Buccini, G. D. S., Pérez-Escamilla, R., Paulino, L. M., Araújo, C. L., & Venancio, S. I. (2017). Pacifier use and interruption of exclusive breastfeeding: Systematic review and meta-analysis. *Maternal & Child Nutrition*, *13*(3). https://doi.org/10.1111/mcn.12384.

20 Hermanson, Å., & Åstrand, L. L. (2020). The effects of early pacifier use on breastfeeding: A randomised controlled trial. *Women and Birth*, *33*(5), e473–e482. https://doi.org/10.1016/j.wombi.2019.10.001.

CHAPTER 4

Feeding Factors that Can (and Do) Affect Sleep

BURPING

Burping is an important tool to help your baby take efficient, effective, and full feedings. I am frequently asked, "How do I burp my baby?" Parents are often afraid they're going to break their baby, but babies aren't as fragile as you might think. To get a good burp, you need to be pretty firm as you're patting his back. Use your hand to rub his back, with alternating pats. Make sure to place your baby high enough on your shoulder or lean him forward on your hand. Your hand should be carefully positioned under his chin, always protecting his airway. You'll never be wasting your time when working on getting a good burp. It's important to attempt to burp before a feed, during a feed, and after a feed. Quick tip: If it's 2:00 a.m. and you've just fed your baby but can't get a burp, lay him flat for a minute or two, then pick him back up and burp again. I'm betting you'll get that burp!

Sometimes you're so exhausted in the middle of the night that you get frustrated trying to burp your baby. You put him back to bed without getting a good burp. Fifteen minutes later the baby is squirming around in the crib as if he's hungry again. You think, "What the hell is going on? I just fed you!"

It's the burp! I promise, the burp is the culprit. Either your baby's belly was hurting because he needed to burp, or he fell asleep and still needed to burp. Once he finally burped, he had more room in his belly to take in more milk—so he's hungry again!

Burping is underrated. It's definitely worth the effort.

REFLUX

Let's talk about reflux. I know a lot of parents worry about gas and reflux, and they think their baby is struggling with sleep because of it. True reflux is most likely not the cause of unexplained crying, irritability, or distress in an otherwise healthy baby. Many first-time parents don't realize that crying can be a normal part of infancy. If it *is* reflux, medication is not the "go to" method for treating babies.[21] The benefits often do not outweigh the risks. There are other more effective treatment options. Do you know what the preferred treatment is? Smaller, more frequent feeds and paced bottle-feeding.[22] Specific burping techniques and being mindful of pressure on your baby's stomach can also help with reflux. Pro tip here: Don't put your baby in her car seat after feeding without getting a good burp. If you do, when you tighten the strap, that bottle's coming right back up.

There are a lot of factors that can contribute to reflux. For

---

21 Alderton, A., & Toop, L. (2012). Irritable Infants, Reflux and Acid Suppression A connection that should never have been made. *Midwifery News, 64*, 18–19.

22 Walls, E. (2019). Understanding reflux problems in infants, children and young people. *British Journal of Nursing, 28*(14), 920.

example, if a mom has a fast letdown or oversupply, her baby might struggle with reflux. A rapid transfer of milk at the breast or bottle can cause reflux. It can be helpful to change to a laid-back position while breastfeeding. If your baby is bottle-feeding, using the paced-bottle technique and correct nipple flow rate is crucial to preventing reflux and promoting infant-led feeding. These two factors can (and do) affect baby's sleep patterns. When a baby is experiencing reflux from being overfed, it affects her sleep. And sometimes when a baby's stomach is hurting from being overfed or needing a good burp, she will give feeding cues. If we immediately feed her without burping or assessing her potential needs, her stomach may continue to hurt. It's important to pay attention to the quality of the feeding and to stop the feeding when your baby is showing signs that she is full.

LAST DAYTIME FEEDING

Many parents reach out to me for nighttime sleep support. They mistakenly think they should give their baby a bottle of formula or pumped breast milk for their last bottle before bed to get their baby to sleep at night. This is not an effective strategy and can be the very reason why their baby isn't sleeping well at night.[23] The baby is forced to take a large volume of milk at the end of the day, which causes an overfed baby to have an uncomfortable stomach.

Recent evidence suggests that human milk is a chrono nutrient that helps infants establish their circadian rhythm.[24] I was excited to find research that supports my experience with a breastfeeding infant. Too many times I've seen recommendations for parents to give pumped

23 Cohen Engler, A., Hadash, A., Shehadeh, N., & Pillar, G. (2012). Breastfeeding may improve nocturnal sleep and reduce infantile colic: Potential role of breast milk melatonin. *European Journal of Pediatrics*, 171(4), 729–732. https://doi.org/10.1007/s00431-011-1659-3.

24 Italianer, M. F., Naninck, E., Roelants, J. A., van der Horst, G., Reiss, I., Goudoever, J., Joosten, K., Chaves, I., & Vermeulen, M. J. (2020). Circadian Variation in Human Milk Composition, a Systematic Review. *Nutrients*, 12(8), 2328. https://doi.org/10.3390/nu12082328.

HILLARY SADLER

breastmilk or formula as the last feeding of the day in order to get their baby to sleep through the night. It is clear that research does not back this recommendation. Remember, your baby will take in different amounts of breast milk or formula at different times of the day. The last feeding of the day will probably be a smaller volume. For breastfeeding and pumping moms, this is especially important to understand. It doesn't matter how much she consumes at which feed. When you set your baby up to take efficient, effective feeds throughout the day, she will learn how to organize her feeds to make up for missed nighttime feedings as she extends her nighttime sleep.

Think about it this way. Most toddlers and preschool children have very small appetites for dinner, but they wake up hungry in the morning and are hungry all day long. My children can eat a 3-course breakfast and then ask for a snack an hour later. They are starving by 4 p.m. But by dinnertime, I'm begging them to please eat at least 3 bites of their dinner. If you keep this in mind when you're feeding your baby, it will help you to feed on cue and worry less about the clock. That being said, I'm not promoting snack feeding. Work on getting your baby to take full feedings at the breast or bottle while also feeding on cue. The ultimate goal is to get him to take in his daily caloric and nutrient needs between the hours of 7 a.m. and 7 p.m., or whatever 12-hour window works best for you.

STARTING SOLIDS

Let's talk about what it looks like to start solids. This book doesn't go into all the details of this topic, but I do want to talk about how solids can affect your baby's routine and nighttime sleep. I've noticed that starting babies on solids between the ages of 6 to 12 months can throw a wrench in their sleep. The reason for this is related to snack feeding.

It's important to offer your baby solids *right after* you breastfeed or bottle feed. It might be the first time you've heard this suggestion, but it's really important. Otherwise, this is what typically happens: Baby takes his liquid feeding, then eats solids an hour later. Then he breastfeeds or bottle-feeds an hour later and goes down for his nap. He didn't do a full liquid feeding because he just ate solids an hour ago, so he wakes up after an hour because he's hungry or thirsty. It becomes a repeated cycle of snack feeding and not getting those quality pockets of sleep. Another potential problem is this: If your baby is filling up on solids throughout the day instead of breast milk or formula, he's going to start waking up at night to get it in. The key point is this: Make sure you couple your breastfeeding or bottle-feeding session with the times you offer solids.

What does this look like in real life? When you breastfeed or bottle-feed, offer your baby solids within 15 to 20 minutes of finishing her liquid feeding. That way she can eat as much as she wants without interfering with her next liquid feeding. And if she doesn't want to eat solids, that's fine. It's a complementary offering. Your baby doesn't need those solids to grow at this point in infancy! Remember, breast milk or formula is your baby's main source of nutrition for the first 12 months of life.

When should you introduce solids into your baby's diet? This is a conversation you should have with your baby's provider, which is typically covered at your 4-month checkup. Some pediatric providers have recently started suggesting solids around the 4-month mark. However, based on current evidence-based research, it's best to wait until your baby is approaching 6 months.[25] Here are some signs to show that your baby might be ready: He is able to sit upright when

25 Papoutsou, S., Savva, S. C., Tornaritis, M., Hadjigeorgiou, C., Hunsberger, M., Jilani, H., Ahrens, W., Michels, N., Veidebaum, T., Molnár, D., Siani, A., & Moreno, L. A. (2018). Timing of solid food introduction and association with later childhood overweight and obesity: The IDEFICS study. *Maternal & Child Nutrition*, 14(1), n/a-1. https://doi.org/10.1111/mcn.12471.

supported and has good head control. More obviously, your baby tries to grab your food and is salivating when watching you eat!

Many parents rush to start solids. Let me tell you something—*don't rush it!* You will save yourself a lot of frustration if you wait until your baby is truly ready. All of my babies were 6 months old before I started solids. They just weren't ready before then. I believe the majority of babies are closer to 6 months old before they're really ready. That being said, refer to your provider about what her recommendation is for starting solids.

ALLERGIES

As we're discussing the introduction of solids, I'd like to mention the subject of allergies. Evidence shows that introducing allergy-triggering foods early on in infancy can actually help desensitize your baby to those allergies.[26] You should expose them to foods such as nuts, eggs, dairy, and strawberries, to name a few. Now, don't go giving your baby a peanut, but you could stir a little bit of peanut butter into his oatmeal.[27]

CHOKING

The last thing I have to say about solids is this: Make sure you know how to respond if your baby chokes. I'm serious. *Take an infant CPR course.* And make sure whoever is watching your child also knows what to do if your baby is choking. I didn't have a serious choking episode until having my third child. She was about 14 months old, sitting upright in her highchair and eating lunch next to my 3-year-old.

26 Anvari, S., Chokshi, N. Y., Kamili, Q. U. A., & Davis, C. M. (2017). Evolution of Guidelines on Peanut Allergy and Peanut Introduction in Infants: A Review. *JAMA Pediatrics, 171*(1), 77–82. https://doi.org/10.1001/jamapediatrics.2016.2552.

27 Burgess, J. A., Dharmage, S. C., Allen, K., Koplin, J., Garcia, L. V., Boyle, R., Waidyatillake, N., & Lodge, C. J. (2019). Age at introduction to complementary solid food and food allergy and sensitization: A systematic review and meta-analysis. *Clinical & Experimental Allergy, 49*(6), 754–769. https://doi.org/10.1111/cea.13.

He was eating a small cracker, and she grabbed one. At first I thought she was going to work it out. She was gagging but then became silent. I could tell she couldn't get it up and couldn't breathe. I went into nurse mode. I grabbed her, patted her on the back for a minute, looked at her and realized, "Oh shit, this is for real." She was still small for a 14-month-old, so I handled her like an infant: I immediately put her face in my hand, directed her head toward the floor and started giving her back blows. I did this 5 times, looked at her, and she was still choking. I thought about my next steps. I gave the back blows one more attempt and was ready to flip her over to start chest thrusts. On the fifth back blow, the small cracker and peanut butter sandwich flew out of her mouth! To say I was relieved doesn't even begin to describe the overwhelming emotion I experienced in that moment. I just broke down crying. I kissed and held her and couldn't believe what had just happened. She was stunned, I was stunned. My 3-year-old was stunned. What if I hadn't been trained as a nurse? What if I didn't know what to do? During that moment my body and mind had automatically shifted into crisis management mode, and I'm so thankful it did. But after the moment was over, I went into mommy mode and just fell apart.

Why am I telling you this? Because if it happens to you, I want you to have a happy ending like I did. Because it may. It's not some far-off possibility. When your child starts eating solids, he could choke. So take a class. Know what to do. If you don't want to sign up at your local hospital, there are many online options to choose from. So just take a class.

Wake

Understand wake windows.

CHAPTER 5

Wake Windows

Wake time. To be completely honest with you, wake time really stressed me out with my first baby. I found myself planning out every minute of wake time. The schedule I was following had it all mapped out for me. I was supposed to make sure my baby had a specific amount of wake time. It was structured. It was stressful. I needed to provide developmentally appropriate toys. It had to happen at a specific time each day. I began to dislike wake time. And the guilt that followed that admission was overwhelming.

Wake time should be time you enjoy. It should be time you look forward to. Imagine what you want your baby's wake time to be. Don't set yourself up for unrealistic expectations. Wake time can simply be sitting on the couch with your baby while you both stare at each other (bring on the baby talk). It can be strapping your baby in a forward-facing baby carrier while you walk around the house organizing or folding laundry. It can be a walk outside in the stroller.

Whatever you want to imagine for wake time for you and your baby, that's what it can be! You don't have to look for activities on Pinterest or have a set schedule for what wake time should look like for your baby. Don't let it stress you out.

THE FIRST 6 WEEKS

During the first 6 weeks of your baby's life there will be very little wake time, and most of that wake time will be feed time. It's important to understand that feeding time is included in wake time. Many babies will close their eyes as they suck on the breast or bottle, but if your baby is actively feeding, this is considered wake time.

Keeping your baby awake for feedings (and wake time) may be one of the most frustrating challenges of the first 6 weeks. It can be a chore. However, it's very important to help your baby have vigorous feeds—to take full feedings during wake time in order to have good pockets of rest between each feeding. And getting good pockets of rest between each wake time is the key to getting your baby to take full feedings. You can see how this cycle can be frustrating.

OVERSTIMULATION

A baby's feed, wake, sleep cycle can easily go off course when she's overstimulated. You can avoid overstimulation by learning your baby's sleepy cues so you know when the wake window should end. If you're following the cues of a newborn (the first 28 days), you'll find that she's unlikely to stay awake for more than 30 minutes at a time. In the first 6 weeks of life, the goal of the wake window is to get full feedings and to keep your baby's world small. Very small. This may be one of the most important things to remember. Understanding this concept will help you keep your baby from becoming overstimulated.

I can't even count the number of times I've walked into a postpartum patient's room to find the parents exhausted and completely overwhelmed. They will report having visitors and interruptions all day long. With the constant changing of arms between friends and family (everyone wants to hold the baby) and hospital policies and procedures requiring constant vital signs, routine tests, and hourly rounds, their baby wasn't able to get good pockets of sleep between each feeding. In the hospital setting, newborn babies often have wake times that extend far beyond the recommended 30-minute window. Before you know it, you have a very unsettled baby who isn't able to feed vigorously and who is very difficult to settle to sleep. This can happen at home too. It's important to break out of this cycle. Prevention is key. You need to limit the wake window to keep your baby from becoming overstimulated.

AFTER 6 WEEKS

After 6 weeks you can start to lengthen your baby's wake window. You will find that wake windows fluctuate throughout the day. Remember how I told you your baby would take in different volumes of breast milk or formula at different feedings throughout the day? The same is true for wake windows. Your baby's magic wake window won't always be 60 minutes. There will be times when she needs to be settled and put to sleep within 45 minutes. At other times, she might make it to 90 minutes. What's most important is to pay attention to your baby's cues.

Here is an example of a typical wake window: Your 8-week-old baby wakes up for her anchor feed after sleeping 9 straight hours during the night. She eats at 7:00 a.m. and goes down for her first nap at 7:45. She sleeps until 10:05—a really good morning nap. She feeds again right away. After her feeding, she is happy, cooing, and interested in interacting with you. She is awake for the full 90-minute wake window then settles back down for her next nap at 11:30 a.m. After about 45 minutes she wakes up happy and ready to go. It's

12:15. She has another feeding and continues in her wake window. But by 1:15 you notice the glazed look in her eye. She yawns. It has only been 60 minutes since she woke up, but you take her to her room and she goes down for her nap immediately. She wakes up again at 3:30 and you start another feed.

This is real life! As you can see, your baby will have different wake periods throughout the day. You cannot hold your baby to a set time frame. If you do, you're likely to have either an understimulated or overstimulated baby.

GROWTH SPURTS

Let's look at growth spurts. When your baby is having a growth spurt, he will be extra hungry. He will feed more frequently, which means he will probably nap for shorter periods in order to wake up and eat. This is normal, and this is good! Every time your baby goes through a growth spurt, he needs to send the message that your body needs to make more milk! This message is delivered by cluster feeding. Your baby has to demand more milk before he gets it. Your body will get the message and make more milk. However, it will take a few days to catch up. For breastfeeding babies, this can throw their "schedule" off. Why? Because they will be hungry! While your body is trying to catch up to his demand, your baby is wanting the groceries now! So, he will wake up early from naps (and nighttime sleep) to get more frequent feeds. As your body adjusts to the increased demand, your baby will take in more volume per feeding, and your good sleeper will return.

I've discussed this before, but I want to emphasize it again because it's critical that you understand this concept: As your baby grows, he will want and need more calories. If you're a breastfeeding mom, your body has to get the message that your baby needs more milk. *Don't hold your baby to the confines of a strict schedule.* I can guarantee that if you do, your breast milk supply will be affected. Any time you start to notice a change in wakefulness, you need to ask yourself, "Is my baby getting enough good, quality feeding sessions?" Increased wakefulness, decreased naps, and decreased nighttime sleep is often related to feeding patterns.

Let's circle back to developmental leaps for a minute. A developmental leap is related to sensory and cognition growth, whereas a growth spurt refers to physical growth. As your baby grows, she becomes more aware of the world around her. When your baby is going through a leap, it's good to be mindful of stimulation during wake windows. She may become overstimulated very easily. During these leaps, go back to making her world small.

THE WITCHING HOUR

The witching hour. It's related to an overstimulated baby and feeding. In an effort to get a good feeding in before bedtime, moms sometimes try to hold off earlier feedings in order to extend their feeding interval in the early evening hours. But guess what? This is not actually helpful at all, especially if you're breastfeeding. Let me explain. Your baby has been feeding at least 8 times per day. Then you start encouraging him to extend his sleep at night. He's growing and gaining weight, and with that his daily caloric requirements are also increasing. Somehow you have to make up the feeds that you're eliminating in the middle of the night. For most babies 12 weeks and younger, especially those that are breastfeeding, they will need to continue to feed at least 6 to 7 times in 24 hours to get the calories they need. So now we only have the hours between 6 a.m. and 9 p.m. to get those feeds in. What does this look like when we map it out? It looks like your baby will be doing some cluster feeding in the evening. Your baby is trying to consume those calories so he can extend his sleep at night. Does it make sense now? When you don't let him get his calories in with clustered feeds, he won't extend his sleep at night because he'll wake up hangry.

What about the overstimulated baby? Remember, overstimulated babies have a hard time falling asleep. By the end of the day, their little brains have had just about all they can take. So it's important to help your baby shut it down and get a cat nap in the evening. This nap could be anywhere from 15 to 60 minutes. But it may have to happen in a baby carrier, swing, stroller, whatever. It's probably not going to happen in the crib.

Here's what I did with my babies, and it worked: Get yourself a baby wrap. I know, they're impossible to figure out how to tie, I agree—but you can watch a YouTube video or the company's website video for a how-to demonstration. It's the best 5 minutes you'll ever spend. It'll save you from the witching hour. So buy your wrap of choice, feed your baby, change her diaper, and then put her in the carrier. Make it part of your routine that she naps in the carrier. I promise, if you're struggling through the witching hour, *this is a game changer*. When your baby wakes up, you can start her bedtime routine, follow it with a feeding, then put her down for the night and treat the remaining feeds as nighttime feeds. Making this your routine each evening will help your baby extend his nighttime sleep. I promise.

The goal of the wake window is to help your baby grow and develop, but you need to be mindful of his current developmental level. If you introduce play or sensory activity that isn't developmentally appropriate, you risk your baby being overstimulated and hard to settle.

Knowing the recommended wake windows based on your baby's age, and following his cues, will help you find the ideal wake period for your baby. However, as much as you try to prevent him from becoming overstimulated, it will happen at some point. What's the answer? Sleep.

FUSSING VS. CRYING

Sometimes babies cry for no reason. This can be unnerving and at times make your skin crawl like fingernails on a chalkboard. When you're feeling maxed out, it's important to take care of yourself as well as your baby. If you reach that point, my advice is to put your baby down in a safe place, take a deep breath, and walk outside for a few minutes.[28]

Crying is normal, but all crying is not the same. As you get to know your baby, you will get to know her cry. Sometimes she just needs to burn off some energy. When babies get overstimulated (sensory overload), crying is their way to deal with it. If your baby has been awake for way longer than her ideal wake window, crying will very likely be her way to fall asleep.

One day I was helping to support a couple with their newborn baby. The mom said, "She is awake all the time. She never goes to sleep." The baby was having weight gain issues, and the pediatrician was worried because she didn't seem to be feeding well. I helped with the feeding, and, as expected, she fell asleep before she could take a full feeding. After some effort, we finally got the baby to take a full feeding. I explained the importance of good pockets of rest between feedings in order to get full feedings each time. Baby girl was so overstimulated that she was having a hard time falling asleep. I swaddled her, placed her on her side (on my lap), and used a tiny jiggle motion to coax her to sleep. She cried frantically for about 2 minutes, and then she was *out*! She slept for 3 hours. It was the longest period of uninterrupted sleep she'd had since coming home from the hospital two weeks prior.

It's not your job to make sure your baby never cries. Sometimes crying is just the thing your baby needs! Your job is to make sure she

28 Wiley, M., Schultheis, A., Francis, B., Tiyyagura, G., Leventhal, J. M., Rutherford, H. J. V., Mayes, L. C., & Bechtel, K. (2020). Parents' Perceptions of Infant Crying: A Possible Path to Preventing Abusive Head Trauma. *Academic Pediatrics*, 20(4), 448–454. https://doi.org/10.1016/j.acap.2019.10.009.

feels loved and secure. When you've addressed all her baby needs (she's been fed and burped, has a clean diaper, there are no hair tourniquets or overly "helpful" siblings) and your baby is still crying, *it is okay.* In this situation, the best thing to do is support your baby's sleep environment and help her get sleep.

What is the difference between fussing and crying? Fussing isn't as intense as crying. And fair warning—fussing will follow your baby into early childhood! But for now, fussing will almost always be your warning sign that your baby is slipping past her optimal wake window.

As you are putting your baby down to sleep after the fussing has started, it's okay if she continues to fuss. Expect it. Letting your baby fuss for a few minutes will not cause her to have attachment issues. In fact, pausing for up to 5 minutes may give her the opportunity to drift to sleep, or back to sleep.

That being said, during the first 3 months of life, it's most important to feed on cue. Pay attention to early feeding cues *before* your baby becomes fussy. For example, if your baby is waking up from sleep and giving you early feeding cues, you don't want to pause for 5 minutes before starting the feeding.

Sleep

Learn how to set your baby up
to sleep through the night.

CHAPTER 6

When Will I Get to Sleep Again?

Getting enough sleep. It's one of the most common fears new moms and dads have (for both their newborn and themselves). It's a legit concern. Evidence-based research confirms that sleep is a priority![29] And you're not alone if you have wondered, "When will I ever get to sleep again?"

After years of working with moms during pregnancy, labor, and postpartum, I've found that most are looking for that one magic solution for getting their baby to sleep through the night. You've likely seen plenty of people claiming to know the trick or secret to getting your little one to do just that. May I share a truth with you? There isn't one.[30]

---

29 Jiang, F. (2020). Sleep and Early Brain Development. *Annals of Nutrition & Metabolism*, 75(Suppl 1), 44–54. https://doi.org/10.1159/000508055.

30 Connell-Carrick, K. (2006). Trends in Popular Parenting Books and the Need for Parental Critical Thinking. *Child Welfare*, 85(5), 819–836.

UNDERSTANDING THE *WHY*

There just isn't a magical trick out there. The truth is, every baby is unique. Your baby's needs aren't the same as my baby's needs. I have good news though: the key to helping your little one extend his night-time sleep is understanding the why behind the all the information, suggestions, quick tricks, and tips that are so readily available.[31] This takes a little time and effort. It looks less like sticking to a schedule and more like taking the time to be properly informed about infant sleep cycles and realistic expectations about naturally extending sleep time. It means implementing the right steps to build a good foundation for sleep, based on your understanding of the research. This approach will help you both get that restorative sleep you crave!

Many parents think "sleep training" is some kind of developmental milestone you have to walk through with your baby. It doesn't have to be. Gaining an understanding about each of these topics and incorporating some foundational practices from day one will help your baby to naturally extend her sleep from 5-6 hours to 6-8 hours, and then to 10-12 hours.[32] The "cry it out" method might sound like an easy approach to sleep training for now, but it doesn't set you up for success in the long run.

How can you feel confident in your ability to figure out what your nonverbal baby needs when no one has taken the time to help you understand the *why* behind their recommendations? *The Feed, Wake, Sleep and Have a Settled Baby Method* does just that.

31 Covington, L. B., Patterson, F., Hale, L. E., Teti, D. M., Cordova, A., Mayberry, S., & Hauenstein, E. J. (2020). The contributory role of the family context in early childhood sleep health: A systematic review. *Sleep Health: Journal of the National Sleep Foundation.* https://doi.org/10.1016/j.sleh.2020.11.010.

32 Douglas, P. S., & Hill, P. S. (2013). Behavioral sleep interventions in the first six months of life do not improve outcomes for mothers or infants: a systematic review. *Journal of Developmental and Behavioral Pediatrics* : JDBP, 34(7), 497–507. https://doi.org/10.1097/DBP.0b013e31829cafa6.

Here are some proven ways to help meet your baby's needs:[33]

- Feeding on cue (whether breast or bottle)
- Hitting "reset" when your baby gets overstimulated
- Following a routine (not a schedule)
- Limiting your baby's wake windows
- Structuring naps
- Properly soothing your baby

THE TRUTH ABOUT SCHEDULES

Many factors come into play when it comes to your baby and sleep. A well-meaning friend might share a "foolproof schedule" with you. But the truth is, you don't want your life being trapped by your baby's schedule. Your baby is constantly changing! Babies go through growth spurts, developmental leaps, teething, illness, you name it. You'll go on vacations, visit your neighbors, stay with your parents—and you'll need the confidence to know what to do without referring to your book, app, or manual every time something happens outside of your "schedule." When you understand the *why*, you can establish a routine you are comfortable with rather than a schedule you hope you can stick to.

SLEEPING THROUGH THE NIGHT

Beware of unrealistic expectations. During the first 6 weeks of your baby's life you will be getting pockets of sleep. Your baby will not sleep through the night. Now, what does "sleeping through the night" even mean? If you ask 5 different people, you will probably get 5 different answers. In this book, if I make reference to sleeping through the night, I mean having *at least 8 hours of uninterrupted sleep.* Eight hours of sleep. If you have a unicorn baby who is sleeping

---

33 Black, M. M., & Aboud, F. E. (2011). Responsive feeding is embedded in a theoretical frame-work of responsive parenting. *The Journal of Nutrition, 141*(3), 490–494. https://doi.org/10.3945/jn.110.129973.

through the night before 6 weeks, don't tell your friends! In all seriousness, having realistic expectations about sleep will help you celebrate your pockets of sleep!

Your baby should not be allowed to sleep longer than a 4-hour stretch until she is back to her birth weight and at least 2 weeks old. If your baby is still asleep as she approaches 4 hours from the start of her last feeding, it's best to wake her so she can feed. Once your baby has passed her birth weight and she's at least 2 weeks old, your pediatric provider will most likely encourage you to let your baby sleep at night until she wakes up on her own. Realistically, during the first 6 weeks of your baby's life you can encourage her to have pockets of sleep that last between 3 to 5 hours at a time. At around week 7, your baby may start to extend her nighttime sleep to 8 hours and will indeed be sleeping through the night. By using *The Settled Baby Method,* you can expect your baby to consistently sleep through the night by 12 weeks old.

THE FEED, WAKE, SLEEP CYCLE

How do you set your baby up for success to be able to sleep through the night by the end of the fourth trimester? It's really simple: Master *The Feed, Wake, Sleep and Have a Settled Baby Method.*

Let's talk more about how sleep is an important part of this method. The first step to setting your baby up for nighttime sleep is to implement the feed, wake, sleep cycle. First and foremost, whenever your baby wakes up from sleep, feed him. This is critical, because your baby will take the fullest feedings immediately following a sleep cycle. There will be times when your baby wakes up and it has only been 30 minutes since the last feeding. It doesn't matter—feed him. Trust me. You don't want to be feeding your baby at the end of a wake window. When you do, your baby will fall asleep and will have taken a snack feed instead of a full feeding.

Earlier I talked about snack feeding and the overstimulated baby, and how this cycle can affect sleep. How do you get your baby out of this cycle? It's really a simple answer. You hit "reset." When you find that your baby is in this cycle, I want you to help your baby get a good nap—a good pocket of rest—no matter where it happens. You may have to do this for a few feeding cycles until your baby is able to take full feedings followed by restful sleep.

Other variables can affect sleep. If you're breastfeeding, remember that your available supply fluctuates throughout the day. There may be times when your baby is ready to eat closer to a 2-hour interval due to your supply and the time of day. It doesn't mean you have a supply issue. It's just the way the breastfeeding relationship works. If you're breastfeeding and feel that you can't get out of the cycle, then I would strongly encourage you to reach out to a local lactation consultant who can help troubleshoot.

Sometimes your baby will be woken up from his slumber before he is ready to wake up. As baby transitions through sleep cycles, sometimes he will seem to wake up but really isn't ready. Here's an example: Grandpa is holding your baby, who just fell asleep 15 minutes ago. Baby starts to stir in Grandpa's arm, and his eyes momentarily pop open. Grandpa starts talking to the baby, stimulating him and waking him up. But he wasn't ready to wake up. What do you do? First, help your baby transition back to sleep by rocking, swaying, swaddling, shushing—whatever you have to do to get your baby back to sleep. Then explain the feed, wake, sleep cycle to Grandpa!

The plan is to feed your baby as soon as he wakes up, but be sure he gets good pockets of sleep. This doesn't mean you have a set period of time when he's supposed to be sleeping. You are supporting his sleep with the ideal sleep environment and letting him wake on his own for feedings (after the first 2 weeks of life and back to birth weight).

How long should your baby be sleeping at night? This will depend on whether he has had organized, efficient, effective feedings during the day. One thing I'd like you to take note of is this: When your baby starts to extend nighttime sleep, he will also start to eat more frequently during the day for a period of time. As your baby grows and takes in more volume per feeding, he will eventually space out his daytime feeds, but it's important to remember that in the beginning, extended nighttime sleep equals more frequent daytime feeds. Essentially, when you take away a nighttime feeding, you need to replace it with a daytime feeding. For breastfeeding babies, this usually happens in the afternoons and evenings.

REASONABLE EXPECTATIONS

Here are reasonable expectations for nighttime sleep (see next chapter on how to adjust your baby's age to the due date):

- Weeks 2-6: Expect a 4-6 hour stretch, then feed every 2-3 hours.
- Weeks 7-12: Expect a 5-10 hour stretch, then feed every 3-4 hours.
- Months 3-5: Expect an 8-12 hour stretch. The goal is to reach 11-12 hours for nighttime sleep. If your baby is sleeping for an 8-hour stretch, feed her, then put her back down for another 3-4 hour stretch.
- Months 6 and beyond: Expect 10-12 hours of uninterrupted sleep.

Helping your baby transition to sleeping through the night does not happen overnight! But now you're better equipped to assess all the factors mentioned in this book that affect nighttime sleep.

CHAPTER 7

Swaddling and Sleep Environment

During the fourth trimester, your baby will need to be soothed. He is not born with the ability to self soothe. And while you want him to learn to soothe himself—and he will—your primary goal in the fourth trimester is to help your baby get good quality sleep and not be continually overstimulated.

By following the guidelines in this book, you *will* have a baby who is able to self soothe. Using a swaddle will be one of the tools to help your baby get good pockets of sleep as well as learn how to self soothe.

SWADDLING

Swaddling. Is it *really* necessary? I've often heard new parents say, "My baby hates to be swaddled." While I would question their statement, I can see why they make it. A lot of people think swaddling means having your baby's arms pinned down to her side as if in a straitjacket. I've seen some well-known sleep consultants recommend this technique, though I disagree with this type of swaddling. In fact, it's not backed by current evidence-based research.[34]

Many babies prefer to have their arms midline to their body. They also need to be free to move their legs up and down and side to side. Have you ever watched your baby lift her legs up and them slam them down? Maybe she is having gas pains. Remember when you were a kid and your stomach hurt? What did you do? Most likely you'd lie on your side or stomach with your kneels pulled up to your chest, assuming the fetal position. Now imagine if you were positioned flat on your back with your arms pinned down by your side. Frustrating, right?

It's important to find the *right* swaddle for your baby! The right swaddle will change based on their age. For example, the little square swaddle blanket the hospital provides is perfect for the first 24 to 72 hours of life. Your baby basically does nothing but eat and sleep. But once you get home, that swaddle probably isn't going to cut it! Your baby becomes a little more wiggly and is often busting out of the swaddle that worked so perfectly in the hospital. Sure, the nurses were "professional swaddlers," but you're a good swaddler too! It's just that your baby has moved past that swaddle.

I wonder how much money parents spend on swaddles. It's a huge market, that's for sure. And all the brands promise that *their* swaddle will help your baby sleep through the night. Swaddling can, and will, help your baby sleep longer periods at night,[35] but as you know, it's not the only factor. When you've addressed all of the other potential reasons you're having issues with your baby sleeping, it's time to

34   Nelson, Antonia, RNC-MNN, PhD & CNE, IBCLC. (2017). Risks and Benefits of Swaddling Healthy Infants: An Integrative Review. MCN, *American Journal of Maternal Child Nursing*, 42, 216-225. https://doi.org/10.1097/NMC.0000000000000344.

35   Möller, E. L., de Vente, W., & Rodenburg, R. (2019). Infant crying and the calming response: Parental versus mechanical soothing using swaddling, sound, and movement. *PLoS ONE*, 14(4), 1.

consider your baby's sleep environment. Having the right swaddle or sleep sack can definitely affect their ability to get good quality sleep! So, let's talk more about swaddles.

When your baby's arms float out in space and startle, he feels like he's falling. Not fun, right? While it is important to let your baby move freely at times, when it's time for sleep he needs to feel secure. This will help to ensure good quality sleep. Learning to self soothe during the first 12 weeks of life will be difficult for your baby if he is constantly feeling like he's falling.

I prefer not to use loose blankets to swaddle for nighttime sleep. I was always concerned about my baby busting out of the swaddle and having a loose blanket in his crib while I was fast asleep. And though I would consider myself a "swaddling pro," sure enough, my babies always busted out of the swaddles. However, blankets can be used to swaddle your baby when you're watching them. Any time you're holding your baby for a nap, a swaddle blanket is appropriate!

Let's take a minute to discuss swaddling during the daytime hours. I've had many parents ask, "Do I need to swaddle my baby for daytime sleep?" Yes. The purpose of a swaddle is to help your baby get good quality pockets of sleep. Whether daytime or nighttime, whenever you put your baby down for a nap, it's helpful to swaddle.

You might be wondering which swaddle is best. I could list my favorite swaddles, but most likely these will quickly become outdated. Thankfully, there are many options to choose from. Here are some things to consider when selecting the right swaddle:

- Baby's arms can be midline to his body.
- The fabric is stretchy but secure.
- A zipper is provided for 2 a.m. feedings!

How long should you swaddle your baby? A hard and fast rule is to swaddle until he's rolling over. This typically happens from 10 to 14 weeks. Once your baby has started to roll to his side, he will most likely be rolling over soon. It is not safe for your baby to sleep swaddled once he is rolling over.

Many babies prefer to sleep on their belly once they learn how to roll from back to front. If your baby is able to roll from her back to her belly, then it is safe for her to sleep on her belly.[36] Let me clarify: It is *not* safe to place your baby on her belly to sleep. But if she can roll to her belly once she's been placed on her back, *then* it is safe for her to sleep on her belly.

How do you transition your baby out of the swaddle? There are many thoughts and suggestions on how to do this. You will see ads for magic sleep suits or other sleep sacks to help your baby transition out of the swaddle. The problem many babies have when going from a swaddle to freedom is the fact that they can no longer "feel their edges." There really isn't a magic trick to this transition. In fact, it really has to do with your baby's developmental level. At around 3 months, the startle reflex will start to disappear. Once it's gone, your baby will be developmentally ready to sleep without being swaddled. That being said, I will share that I found the *Zipadee Zip* to be very helpful with this transition. My babies could still feel their edges while having the freedom to move around and sleep on their belly if they wanted to (all of my babies were belly sleepers as soon as they learned to roll).

---

36 Adams, S. M., Ward, C. E., & Garcia, K. L. (2015). Sudden infant death syndrome. *American Family Physician, 91*(11), 778–783.

SLEEP ENVIRONMENT

Here are a few more things to consider as it pertains to your baby's sleep environment:

- Make sure it's cool but not cold. A comfortable temperature will promote better sleep.

- Use a sound machine. Turn it to the white noise option and turn up the volume.

- Keep the room dark. Your baby doesn't need a night light. Blackout curtains are strongly recommended.

- Sleep sacks are not all created equal. If your baby is in a sleep suit/sack that doesn't allow him to roll onto his belly, this could affect sleep.

CHAPTER 8

Setting Baby Up to Sleep

MYTHS

I've helped many exhausted parents get some much-needed sleep by busting myths they've heard from well-meaning family or friends. It usually goes something like this: "You shouldn't swaddle your baby during the day," or "Sound machines are only for nighttime sleep." Wrong and wrong. Any time your baby is sleeping, the goal is for your baby to get good pockets of restorative sleep, then to wake up and take a good feeding. During the first 12 weeks, your baby will take many naps throughout the day. If you're holding your baby or carrying her in a wrap, a stroller, or a car seat, you don't need to swaddle her. But when your baby is sleeping independently for any nap, she should be swaddled or in an age-appropriate sleep sack. Support your baby's sleep by creating the optimal sleep environment, whether daytime or nighttime.

NAPS

The next consideration in extending nighttime sleep are daytime naps. Daytime naps promote nighttime sleep. The suggestions I share include the times of day I recommend putting your baby down for a nap. Please keep in mind, you can't be a prisoner in your home so that your baby gets his daytime nap in his crib *every day*. It's just not realistic. But generally speaking, the goal is to get two good naps in his crib whenever possible. It's really important to follow the anchor feed with a good nap in the crib. If your baby takes a good morning nap, you will notice that your entire day seems to go a little better. Ideally the midday nap that follows the lunch feed also happens in the crib. That's really it! The other naps can happen on the go.

A little more about daytime naps. Most babies won't transition into a set nap schedule until about 4 months old. Why? Because of the frequency of feeds during the day. This is especially important to understand as you encourage your baby to transition to extended nighttime sleep. Remember, when your baby starts to extend his sleep at night, he will feed at closer intervals throughout the day. This prevents him from taking extended naps during the day. But once your baby is over 4 months old and his stomach has grown, he will probably take larger volumes per feed. This means you will do fewer feeds in a 24-hour period.

My tip is to go with the flow. Follow the suggested routine, making sure to feed on cue. This will encourage your baby to extend his nighttime sleep.

NAP DURATION

Here are some recommendations and *realistic expectations* for nap durations based on your baby's age. These are approximations. Let your baby nap during the day until he wakes on his own (unless he's sleeping past a 3½ hour feeding interval).

For example: If your baby eats at 9 a.m. and goes down for a nap at 10:15, you should wake her at 12:30 p.m. for a feeding if she is still sleeping.

- Birth to 12 weeks: (5 naps) 30-120 minutes per nap

- 3 to 4 months: (3-5 naps) 30-120 minutes per nap

  Your baby will take shorter naps if he's taking 4-5 naps per day. During the 4th month, try to transition to 3 naps, with the third one lasting only about 45 minutes.

- 5 to 6 months: (2-3 naps) 45-120 minutes per nap

  If your baby takes a short morning or after-lunch nap, you may need to offer a 3rd short nap in the early evening to help her make it to the evening bedtime/feeding routine. The goal is to prevent your baby from becoming overstimulated.

- 7 to 15 months: (2 naps) 30-180 minutes per nap

  The morning nap may last only 30 to 60 minutes. The after-lunch nap should be the primary nap of the day, hopefully lasting at least 90 minutes. If your baby is sleeping longer in the morning and waking early from her after-lunch nap, you may need to limit the duration of the morning nap to 30 to 45 minutes.

- 15 months to 4+ years: (1 nap) 90-120+ minutes

  If your baby doesn't nap well during the day, feed her and put her to bed earlier in the evening. Remember, overstimulated babies have a harder time transitioning to sleep and staying asleep. On the busy days that seem to fall apart, put your baby to bed 30 to 45 minutes early to promote extended nighttime sleep.

CHAPTER 9

Tools to Promote Sleep

ROCKING TO SLEEP

Let's talk about some common concerns parents have related to sleep props. Many worry that holding or rocking their baby to sleep will forever doom them to not being able to sleep through the night. During the first 3 months, it is okay to help your baby transition into a deep sleep before putting him down. Rocking can absolutely be a part of your bedtime routine! I rocked all of my babies and enjoyed the snuggles. On the really busy days, it helped fill up their little love tanks. Ideally, I put them down when drowsy but still awake, but sometimes that didn't happen. If your baby gets overstimulated or is going through developmental leaps or an illness, he may need help transitioning to deep sleep before being put down in order to stay asleep. Rocking is one of your tools to reset your baby's sleep.

THE FIVE S'S

Using the five S's to help your baby transition to sleep is appropriate during the first 12 weeks of your baby's life (remember to adjust age for preterm babies) and any time your baby gets overstimulated. The five S's are: swaddle, side or stomach (when on lap), shush, swing, and suck. These are all helpful tools to calm a crying baby.

LAST DAYTIME FEEDING

Breastfeeding your baby right before putting her to bed for the night can be very beneficial. The comfort baby experiences when nursing helps her get ready for nighttime sleep.

Some people recommend that breastfeeding moms give a bottle at the last feed of the day instead of breastfeeding. I don't recommend this, unless it is what you want to do. You don't have to give a bottle before bed in order to get your baby to sleep through the night. And as I said, if you're primarily breastfeeding, your baby may not get the comfort from the bottle that she gets from breastfeeding; in fact, it may have the opposite effect. One exception: If your baby isn't getting her daily calorie needs at the breast throughout the day, this can affect nighttime sleep. But in general, problems with extending sleep at night are not because she's breastfeeding for the last feed of the day.[37]

PACIFIERS

What about pacifiers to help with nighttime sleep? Some babies love them, others don't. Sucking on a pacifier *can* help soothe a baby to sleep. If using a pacifier, I recommend taking it out of the baby's mouth after he's asleep. However, then he won't be able to find the paci when it falls out of his mouth, so there's that to consider. [38]

37 Barry, E. S. (2020). What Is "Normal" Infant Sleep? Why We Still Do Not Know. *Psychological Reports*, 33294120909447. https://doi.org/10.1177/0033294120909447.

38 Byars, K. C., & Simon, S. L. (2017). American Academy of Pediatrics 2016 Safe Sleep Practices: Implications for Pediatric Behavioral Sleep Medicine. *Behavioral Sleep Medicine, 15*(3), 175.

Parents often worry about their baby getting hooked on a paci and then having a hard time taking it away. Let me share my experience with you: My middle child was about 8 months old and using a pacifier. You know the green ones they give you in the hospital? You can also buy them in stores. Well, they very clearly say "zero to three months," but I never paid attention to the packaging. I was putting my baby down for a nap, and I heard a squeak. He was sucking on his paci. I pulled it out of his mouth, and he had bitten the tip of it. The tip was hanging on by a thread! You can imagine my response. I threw the paci across the room and started crying. *What if my baby had swallowed the plastic tip and choked while he was napping?* Choking is silent. I wouldn't have heard anything on the monitor. Do you know what I did? I put him down for a nap without a paci, endured some crying, and found every paci we owned and chucked them in the trash. I even recruited my 4-year-old to help me. We never looked back. My point is this: Make sure you pay attention to the age range recommendations for the pacifier, and don't make getting rid of it more of a big deal than it is. If you use a paci, great. When you're done, just be done with it. It doesn't need to be a big, hyped-up process of weaning your child from the pacifier.

One more thing I'd like to mention. If your baby has relied on sleep aids for the first 3-4 months of his life, such as a newborn lounger, a crib or bassinet with automatic vibrating, swinging, or swaying motion, or co-sleeping, it might be a little more of a challenge helping your baby to get uninterrupted sleep once you've transitioned away from those aids.

During the first 12 weeks of life, there will be times when your baby truly needs your help to transition to sleep. I recommend starting with the five S's. During this time you're laying the foundation for your baby to learn how to self soothe and transition to sleep without the use of sleep aids. And again, it's ideal to put your baby to bed awake, but drowsy, at least 80 percent of the time. Let her try to fall asleep on her own. Later, you'll learn to help your baby transition to self-soothing if she is still having difficulties after the first 3 months.

Have a Settled Baby

You've got this!

CHAPTER 10

Getting More Sleep

ESTABLISHING A ROUTINE

Let's have a heart-to-heart conversation. You want to establish a routine. You want to get some sleep. It's probably the main reason you're reading this book, right? You want me to give you the magic trick to get your baby to sleep through the night. I totally get it. I am a type A personality, and I *do not* function well with little sleep. With each of my children, during the weeks leading up to their birth, I experienced major anxiety thinking about the lack of sleep I would soon be getting. I'm sure I'm not alone. A lot of parents worry about it, *and rightly so*! I would love to be able to say something comforting like, "Don't worry, your baby will sleep," but that wouldn't be truthful, and I'm committed to telling you the truth.

It really *is* important to start laying the foundation for good sleep habits during the newborn period. It can make sleep training so much easier down the road. The current evidence- based research shows that it's best to wait until your baby is at least 4 to 6 months old to implement behavioral strategies like the "cry it out" method.[39] And that's what you will see me promoting here.

So, what can you do from Day 1 to help with sleep? There are countless methods and books written to help parents extend their baby's sleep, but again, the *why* is missing. They give you a schedule and say, "Here, figure it out." But it's never as simple as that.[40] You need to understand *why* your approach to feeding and wake time is setting your baby up for sleep. This will give you the confidence you need to troubleshoot and know when to be flexible. *The Settled Baby Method* will help you to make the best choices for your baby and yourself as you develop a beneficial routine.

There is no argument as to whether or not sleep is important. We all agree, it's the best thing for parents and baby! Babies need uninterrupted sleep appropriate for their age and developmental level. It is true that some babies are better sleepers than others, but implementing some foundational techniques to promote sleep will feel natural, not a "thing" you have to train your baby to do.

So, how does sleep relate to a daily routine? During infancy, one of the purposes of a routine is to help organize your baby's sleep pockets, facilitate quality playtime for developmental opportunities, give his little belly some "rest time" between feeds to help support his immature GI tract, and to help *you* plan your day. This is possible because there is a flow to your baby's day that you can count on. It helps you to be in tune with what your baby really needs when he's crying but unable to verbalize it. It allows you to get some quality

---

39 Leach, P. (2015). Controlled Crying: What parents need to know. *International Journal of Birth & Parent Education*, 2(4), 13–17.

40 Harries, V., & Brown, A. (2019). The association between baby care books that promote strict care routines and infant feeding, night-time care, and maternal-infant interactions. *Maternal & Child Nutrition*, 15(4), e12858. https://doi.org/10.1111/mcn.12858.

sleep, which, in turn, helps you to be a better parent.[41] Having a routine is not about adhering to a rigid, unrealistic schedule that is more stressful than if you had just followed your baby's cues.

THE 80/20 PRINCIPLE

I want to say something about my own experience with schedules: With my first child, I was the mom who followed the book schedule *to the letter*. And it was hell. Listen to me—the routine I am promoting is your ticket to *thrive* during infancy, not just survive! I like to think of my baby routine like I think of my diet—80/20. Yes, 80/20 is the way to go. You don't want to be so scheduled that you're missing out on life! We all need some spontaneity! If you follow your routine 80 percent of the time, along with the tips you've learned, your baby will sleep! If you go on vacation for a week, you can get back into your routine when you get home. Life is too short to be limited by a strict feeding and sleeping schedule.

RECOMMENDED ROUTINES

I'm going to share my recommended routines with you to use as a guide. Let them guide you into a routine that works for your family. There are specific times listed, but they are *not* meant for you to follow verbatim. They are just a reference.

If you want to start your day at 6 a.m., do it! If you want to start your day at 8 a.m., do it. Then adjust your routine according to the time you want to start. My husband and I like to have our kids in bed by 7 p.m. so we can have some time to ourselves. Our goal, after 4 to 6 months, is to have our baby sleeping 10 to 12 hours at night with no interruptions.

---

41 Kingsley, K., Sagester, G., & Weaver, L. L. (2020). Interventions Supporting Mental Health and Positive Behavior in Children Ages Birth--5 Yr: A Systematic Review. *American Journal of Occupational Therapy, 74*(2), 1–29. https://doi.org/10.5014/ajot.2020.039768.

Let's look at the routine for baby's first 2 weeks. You have three important steps to follow:

1. Feed your baby on cue.[42] It doesn't matter if your baby is breastfeeding or bottle-feeding—feed her on cue. That means feeding every 1½ to 3½ hours with possibly a 4-hour stretch at night.

2. Follow the feed, wake, sleep cycle as closely as possible. Feed, followed by a short period of wake time (15 to 20 minutes), followed by sleep.

3. If your baby gets overstimulated and it's been more than 2 hours since she went to sleep, do whatever you can to get your baby to sleep. Use any of the sleep aids that work for you to help your baby "reset" and get back on track. Remember the five S's: swaddling, side-lying or belly position (while being held), shushing, sucking, and swinging.

This is it. This is all you need to do during the first 2 weeks as it relates to sleep. Remember, your baby shouldn't sleep more than 4 hours at a time during the first 2 weeks of life. As you can see, during this time, you can realistically only expect to get pockets of broken sleep.

ANCHOR FEED

What is our plan after the first 2 weeks? I'm glad you asked! It's much of the same, but we're going to start anchoring the first morning feeding. This means that you will choose a time to start each day. For example, if you start your day at 7 a.m., that is your anchor feed. You'll feed your baby within 30 minutes of 7 a.m. every day. This is one of the most important parts of your routine. Your anchor feed is your foundation. It will encourage a consistent flow, or rhythm, to your days.

Here's an example: My baby's anchor feed is at 7 a.m. She wakes up at 5:30 for a feeding. I feed her *as if it's a nighttime feeding*, then put her back to sleep for the rest of the night. I wake her up by 7:30 for

42   Chen, T. L., Chen, Y. Y., Lin, C. L., Peng, F. S., & Chien, L. Y. (2020). Responsive Feeding, Infant Growth, and Postpartum Depressive Symptoms During 3 Months Postpartum. *Nutrients, 12*(6), 1766. https://doi.org/10.3390/nu12061766.

her anchor feed, even though she just ate at 5:30. She probably won't eat as much because she just ate 2 hours ago, but the rest of the day will have a predictable flow. This anchor feed will set her up for the rest of the day. Now, what if she wakes up at 6:20? I would feed her and count that as my anchor feed because it's only 10 minutes off of my goal. Ideally, I would try to wait until 6:30 to feed, but I wouldn't allow her to get upset and frantic while waiting.

After your anchor feeding, enjoy interacting with your baby during wake time. Be sure to pay attention to cues that tell you your baby is tired. She might yawn, rub her eyes, avoid eye contact, or start to fuss. When your baby is less than 6 weeks old, it could be just 45 minutes after she wakes up. It's important to put her down awake and tired, but not overtired. An overtired baby will have a harder time falling asleep.

As soon as your baby wakes up, feed her. During the first 3 months of life, it doesn't matter what time she wakes up—feed her. If she is extending her feeding intervals longer than $3\frac{1}{2}$ hours during the day, then she might not be able to fit in all her feeds, causing a nighttime feeding to occur. So if she's still asleep at the $3\frac{1}{2}$ hour mark, I would wait 10 to 15 minutes more and then wake her up, because she needs to eat.

Remember, it's best to have your baby take her morning and midday nap in her crib if possible. The other naps can happen on the go. The evening nap is important for nighttime sleep because it helps the last feeding of the day to be vigorous and, hopefully, a really good feeding. Try to make this evening nap happen, and use whatever technique you need to get your baby to nap. Don't forget the tips I shared earlier about evening naps. In my house, evening naps happened in my fabric baby wrap while I was cooking dinner or folding laundry. (At 6 to 8 months, your baby will probably drop the cat nap. At that point, your bedtime will move up about an hour.)

After the evening nap, it's time to start your bedtime routine. The goal is to keep stimulation to a minimum and get your baby to associate the routine with bedtime. Before starting the next feeding, change her diaper and put her in her sleep outfit. After the feed, place her right in the crib. The last daytime feeding will be between 6:30 and 8 p.m., depending on your routine. *Any subsequent feedings are considered nighttime feeds until the next day's anchor feed.* Be sure to limit stimulation during nighttime feeds. Don't feed your baby in front of the TV or turn all the lights on. Use as little light as you can. Before you start the feeding, I recommend changing her diaper without talking too much. After feeding, your baby will go right back to sleep. Keep nighttime feeding as boring as possible—you don't really want your baby fully waking up. You may have heard this feed described as a "dream feed."

A note for breastfeeding moms. Nighttime feeds can be hard—I know! I was always worried about falling asleep while feeding my baby. Here's a tip: Set your phone alarm for 15 minutes. That way, if you do fall asleep, you're assured that you'll wake up. I did this in the early days of breastfeeding, and it helped a lot. The alarm almost never went off because I was awake, but it gave me peace of mind so I could relax during nighttime feedings. Another tip: If your baby is having a hard time going to sleep at night, it could be because she is overstimulated at the end of the day. Bump the bedtime up 15 or 30 minutes.

Here is an example: A family with a 10-month-old baby was having difficulty with nighttime sleep. As we were troubleshooting, I noticed a possible contributing factor—the baby was staying up until 8 p.m. with her big sister. Once we bumped her bedtime up to 6:30 p.m., she transitioned to sleeping 12 hours at night!

Before you start transitioning to the recommended routines, I want to make sure you understand how to make the routine work for your baby. Remember, if she is hungry, feed her. We talked about it earlier, but I want to state it again: *There is no point in holding your baby off for feeds.* If you're not physically in the right space to feed your baby (driving a car, in a grocery store, on a walk), then, of course, holding your baby off for a feeding is fine. I'm referring to the times when your baby wakes up hungry from a nap but it's not "time" to feed her; or she doesn't want to go down for a nap like she usually does, and your gut feeling is that she's hungry. Feed her. The recommended routines are only a guide—it is always okay to add in an extra feeding.

WEEKS 2-6

Let's look at a routine for 2 to 6 weeks: You are breastfeeding your baby at 3:30 p.m. and a nap is to follow at 4:30. You've tried every trick you know to get your baby to sleep, but she won't fall asleep. Your gut is telling you that she's hungry. Your routine suggests a nap between the 3:30 and 5:30 feeding, but that isn't happening. So what do you do? Instead of trying to hold her off for the 5:30 feeding, go ahead and feed her at 5:00. Instead of an hour of wake time, put her right down for a nap since she skipped the last one. Instead of her 4:30 nap, you fed her instead, which was the right thing to do. So now she's taking her 6:30 nap early. Once she wakes up from this nap, start the quick bedtime routine and feed her the last daytime feeding, which typically happens between 7 and 8 p.m. Being flexible with your evening routine allows your baby to cluster her feedings together in the evening, which will help her extend her nighttime sleep.

Let's talk about the 10 to 11 p.m. feeding during the first 6 to 8 weeks. Your recommended routine suggests waking your baby for this feeding, which is appropriate about 80 percent of the time. However, there is another option if your baby hasn't been feeding vigorously at this feeding. Here is a personal example: My baby Ruth never fed well when I woke her for this feeding. She would cluster feed every 60 to 90 minutes between the hours of 4 and 6:30 and then be ready for bed by 7 p.m. every night. I would wake her up between 10 and 11 p.m. to feed her, but she wouldn't feed well. It didn't matter whether she was breastfeeding or bottle-feeding—she wanted to be asleep. Soon she'd wake up again between midnight and 1 a.m. ready to feed. After a full, vigorous feeding she'd go right back to sleep for another 3 to 4 hours. It was really difficult for me to wake up for the 10 to 11 p.m. feeding. I would often go to sleep at about 7:30, and it was so much harder for me to wake up at 10 p.m. as opposed to the 12 to1 a.m. feeding. Then I realized that waking Ruth for the 10 to 11 p.m. feeding was pointless. It was more like a snack feed. So I changed my routine. The next night I put her to bed after her 6:30 p.m. feeding and let her sleep until she woke up. I got a full 7 hours of sleep for the first time since her birth, and she wasn't even 6 weeks old! She slept until 2 a.m. and had extended her feeding interval 7½ hours. It would have been nice to get the 7½ hour stretch after the 10 p.m. feeding, but Ruth was too sleepy to feed well during the first half of the evening. By letting her sleep until she was ready to wake up and feed (after the 6:30 p.m. feeding), we had gone from 3 to 2 middle-of-the-night feedings. Within a week of making this transition, she started to feed about 10 minutes longer at 2 a.m., which helped her get closer to the morning anchor feed.

By the time Ruth was 8 weeks old, her routine consisted of a last daytime feed at 6:30 p.m., and a middle-of-the-night feeding between 2 and 3 a.m. Her next feeding was her anchor feed at 6:30 a.m.

By 4 months old she was sleeping uninterrupted from 6:45 p.m. to 6 a.m. I'm sharing this with you because I want you to feel confident following your baby's cues. Had I not allowed Ruth to skip the 10 p.m. feeding, it would have taken her much longer to organize her nighttime feedings.

So if you wake your baby to feed at 10 p.m. but find that he is just snacking, try letting him sleep until he wakes on his own to feed.

One last thing I'd like to review before you look at the recommended routines: It is normal for a baby (especially a breastfed baby) to feed more than 8 times in a 24-hour window. The routines help you map out 8 to 9 feedings every 24 hours, but that does not mean you should *only* allow your baby 8 feedings. Remember, when your baby is going through a growth spurt, a developmental leap, or an illness, you may need to feed your baby 9 or 10 times that day (or for a few days). If you're a breastfeeding mom, it is especially important that you let your baby have those extra feedings. Once again, the reason is this: your body needs to get the message that your baby is growing and needing more milk! It takes your body a few days to respond. By holding your baby to a set number of feedings each day, you're potentially creating a breast milk supply issue.

Whether breastfeeding or bottle-feeding, if you're not allowing your baby to feed when he's hungry, you're not helping him to extend nighttime sleep. Remember to feed on cue. If your baby starts waking up early from daytime naps, continue to follow the feed, wake, sleep, feed cycle. If your baby was sleeping 8 hours at night and is now waking up hungry after 4 hours, feed him. He is probably in a growth spurt.

The last thing to say about routines is this: Trust your instinct. All the information I've given you is meant to give you tools to help assess the situation and figure out the root of the problem. The purpose of routines is to assist you in figuring out a plan. Ultimately, you know what's best for your baby.

CHAPTER 11

Sleep Regressions

Don't let sleep regressions throw you off your game. You've got this! It's true, you want your baby to sleep at night because *you* want to sleep at night. I get it. You were used to waking up every 2 to 4 hours in the middle of the night and were kind of okay with it, but then your baby began sleeping longer stretches, and now these middle-of-the-night wakings are like torture. I've been there. You're trying to catch up on all those lost hours of sleep that have accumulated over the past few months, and these wakings seem harder than before. So, let's just start there. You've acknowledged that they are tough, and it's okay that you're looking for a way out of them! I would be too. When your baby starts waking up at night, just look at the big picture and try to figure out what is going on. It could be so many things. And as you know, it's not the same for every baby.

Sleep regressions. I don't want you to assume this will happen. Your baby might just sleep right through it. But I do want to give you some tools to help, and the information you need to assess what's going on with your baby. At about 4 months, sleep regressions can be caused by many variables:

BREASTFEEDING

Believe it or not, breastfeeding can be the culprit. First things first, make sure your baby is getting his *daily* caloric intake needs met. If your baby has started to extend his sleep at nighttime, are you allowing for enough feeds during the day for him to get his calories in?[43] More times than not, this is the issue. Here is an example: Your baby was feeding 7 to 8 times in 24 hours, then you dropped his 2 night feedings. Since he's now only feeding 5 to 6 times in 24 hours, he might not be getting enough calories. Remember, mom's supply can fluctuate throughout the day, so be sure to allow your baby to cluster feed in the evening to make up for the feedings he's dropping at night.

DEVELOPMENTAL LEAPS

Next, consider developmental leaps. Maybe your baby has started rolling over. She is definitely more aware of her environment at 4 months old. If your baby is more distracted during the day and isn't feeding well, then she'll make up for it at night! *So how do you get your baby to feed better during the day?* Try to limit distractions. This might require a dark room for feedings during the day. This is just a transitional phase. You're not doomed to feed in a closet for the rest of infancy. Distractions due to developmental leaps can cause a feeding issue during the daytime, and then your baby will make up for it at night, wanting to feed at times when she used to sleep. *Feed her.* If you know she didn't feed well during the day, then feed her at night! Otherwise, you could start having a supply issue. The next day, hit reset and try to get those good feeds in during the daytime.

43 Bearzatto, A. (2020). Slow weight gain in the breastfed infant. *Breastfeeding Review*, 28(1), 39–46.

TEETHING

Teething can affect how your baby sleeps. Mouth and gum pain can be very distressing, so talk to your baby's provider about helping your baby during this painful time. Be aware that there are many gimmicks out there for teething, and some of them are even harmful. Teething is an unavoidable challenge in your baby's development. Expect it, accept it, and try to deal with it the best you can. It won't last forever. When my babies were teething, they were always a little extra cranky and wanted to be close to me. We added a few extra feedings on days that were really rough because it helped get us out of the cycle of interruptive, non-restorative sleep.

DIAPERS

Diapers and sleep—have you thought about how they're related? Here's a quick tip: Size up at night. Sometimes babies start waking up at night because their diapers are really full and it bothers them. When you aren't doing as many middle-of-the-night feedings and your baby is sleeping 10 to 12 hours at night, he will start filling his diaper up. So size up for nighttime sleep!

STARTING SOLIDS

Starting solids can affect your baby's routine and nighttime sleep. I've noticed with babies between 5 and 12 months, starting solids can throw a wrench in their sleep. The main reason for this is snack feeding. Remember, in order to establish a good sleep routine, it's important to offer your baby solids *right after you breastfeed or bottle feed*. Otherwise, this could happen: Your baby takes his liquid feeding then eats solids an hour later; he won't do a full liquid feeding when it's time for him to go down for his nap because he just ate an hour ago, but he wakes up hungry in an hour. So break the cycle of snack feeding in order to get quality pockets of sleep.

107

HILLARY SADLER

To review: If your baby is filling up on solids instead of breast milk or formula throughout the day, he will start waking up at night to get the breast milk or formula feedings he missed. So be sure to couple your breastfeeding or bottle-feeding session with the times you offer solids. Remember, breast milk or formula is your baby's main source of nutrition for the first 12 months of life.

SLEEP SUPPORT

The last thing I want you to consider when you find yourself in the middle of a sleep regression is this: What type of sleep supporting items are you using? If you went from a swaddle to an arms-out sleep sack, maybe your baby isn't ready for that. Once your baby has grown out of a swaddle, find a sleep sack that is comfortable and secure to help your baby with this transition.

ROOM TEMPERATURE

Is it possible that your baby is feeling too cold at night? When he was swaddled, he was probably a bit warmer having his hands and arms tucked close to his body. Make sure your baby's sleep environment supports sleep. It should be neither too warm nor too cold—72 degrees is just perfect.

To recap, in order to lay the foundation for extending nighttime sleep follow these daily guidelines:

- Anchor the morning feed.
- Get two naps in the crib.
- Make sure baby is getting his calories.
- Take an early evening cat nap (until 6 to 8 months old).

108

CHAPTER 12

My Baby Is Still Not Sleeping

L et's talk about some techniques that will help your baby if she's having issues with sleep, and you've assessed all the things we discussed earlier in the book. You may need to incorporate some behavioral techniques such as allowing your baby to attempt to self soothe in a more structured way, once your baby is at least 4 to 6 months old. I recommend you and your partner work together as a team to help your baby. It can be really hard for one person to be the primary implementer, and it's physically and emotionally exhausting for a few days. Have you ever heard that it takes at least 3 days to break a habit or start a new habit? Keep that in mind if you've determined that your baby's sleep issues are related to behavioral factors and habits that don't promote sleep.

Here is an example: You're traveling. Your baby is sleeping in a portable crib in your room. Being in a new place, your baby wakes up multiple times during the night. You pick her up to assist her back to sleep. I can guarantee that when you've gone past the 3-day threshold with a new sleep "habit," you'll have to help your baby reset into her normal sleep routine. This is to be expected, but I want you to be prepared for it!

GESTATIONAL AGE

Before implementing behavioral techniques to assist your baby with extending nighttime sleep, please review expectations for sleep based on your baby's *adjusted gestational age*: Our benchmark for gestational age is 40 weeks. If your baby is 8 weeks old but was born at 37 weeks gestation (3 weeks early), you need to adjust your baby's age (8 weeks minus 3 weeks) to 5 weeks old. It's important to adjust your baby's age to have realistic expectations for your baby's sleep patterns. When parents do this, very little behavioral modification is needed to assist with extending nighttime sleep.

SLEEP ENVIRONMENT

Keep in mind what you learned about your baby's sleep environment:

- Room temperature: You want the room to be cool. The American Academy of Pediatrics recommends having a circulating fan in your baby's room to promote safe sleep. I agree. I can't tell you how many times I have woken up at night because one of my kids turned my fan off.

- Sound machine: A sound machine is a must-have. I found the white noise option to work best. Be sure to turn the volume up, and check to see that it has batteries in it!

- Blackout curtains: Having blackout curtains can mean the difference between waking up at 5:30 or 7:30 a.m., and let me tell you, that's a big difference! They are obviously helpful with daytime sleep. And in the evening, when it's daylight savings time and your baby goes to bed when it's still light outside, blackout curtains will help him go to sleep more easily.

EARLY WAKING

Let's talk about early morning wakings. They *will* happen. Babies will go through a phase of waking up earlier than we'd like. If your baby is over 6 months old and is starting to wake up earlier than the anchor feed, I have a tip for you. *Don't make this your new wake up time.* If your baby is in her room babbling and not upset, let her work it out—she will be fine.

If you've planned to start your day at 7 a.m. and she's awake right before 6 a.m., leave her in the crib. She'll likely go back to sleep after 30 minutes. It might not happen the first day, but if you don't get her at 5:30 a.m., she'll adjust and stop waking up so early. However, if you do start getting her up—especially if you've done it 3 days in a row—you now have a 6 a.m. alarm clock that'll just keep going off.

Here's a reminder about swaddles and sleep sacks to help your baby sleep. If your baby is less than 3 months old, a swaddle will help him sleep better for daytime and nighttime sleep. Most babies don't like their arms swaddled down by their sides but prefer to have them midline to their body. Babies often like to have their fists up under their chin. The goal of a swaddle is to prevent the startle reflex, which makes babies feel like they are falling. This reflex can wake them up. Find a swaddle that gives your baby options for their arms but prevents the startle reflex.

STRATEGIES FOR CRYING IT OUT

The best way to support your baby to sleep is to follow the foundational methods found in this book. If you are able to implement the suggestions in the first 3 months of your baby's life, you probably won't need to read this section of the book.

If your baby is having trouble extending her nighttime sleep (and is at least 4 to 6 months old), and you've considered all other potential causes, I recommend letting your baby try to work it out and self soothe, starting with 5-minute pockets. Set a timer, because 5 minutes of crying will feel like an hour. As you're trying to help your baby extend her sleep, keep in mind that all the research shows that babies need extended sleep for optimal brain development.

At the 5-minute mark, go into your baby's room but don't talk to her or pick her up. Place your hand on her back or stomach, or help her lie down if she's standing. You're letting her know you're there, but then leave after about a minute. Start the cycle again, but increase the time to 10 minutes. Then the next time wait for 15 minutes before going back into her room. Most babies will go to sleep after about 30 minutes, but you might have a stubborn little one! For nighttime sleep, try to stick with it. If you throw in the towel after an hour, then tomorrow night your baby will protest for at least an hour. Babies are smart!

If you're applying this method for naps during the day, which I highly recommend, then limit the nap time to about 2 hours. If your baby protests for 2 hours and never goes to sleep, get him up, feed him, pay attention to his cues, and repeat at the next nap. If he protests his naps twice in a row, then after the second nap, feed him and hit reset. You'll have to get this nap in wherever you can, because now your baby is probably overtired, and it will be hard to get him to fall asleep in his crib. Remember, the last nap of the day—the one that happens during the witching hour—is not likely going to happen in the crib. Don't try to push that nap in the crib; it's probably a wasted effort.

CLOSING

You can do this! I know this is a lot of information, and much has been repeated to help it sink in. My intention is not to make you an expert about babies and sleep training, but to give you the tools you need to help your baby take efficient, effective feeds and get restorative sleep. I want you to feel comfortable asking your pediatric provider questions that you might not have known to ask prior to reading this book.

What I truly hope for you is this: I hope you do what works best for you and your baby. If my recommended routines and techniques don't work for your family, I hope you will find what does. I want you to gain knowledge and confidence to follow your intuition and put into practice your own assessment skills, based on evidence-based studies, to uniquely care for your baby.

Whether you're breastfeeding or pumping, I hope your journey is better than you imagined. I really do. If it's breastfeeding, that's wonderful. If it's a combination of breastfeeding and supplementing, or exclusively pumping, that's wonderful. If you decide it's best for you and your baby to bottle feed with formula, then that's the best thing to do for your baby! Each of these choices will nurture your baby and help him grow. Yes, the benefits of breast milk can't be ignored, but other important factors go into nurturing our babies as well, which deserve our consideration. My heart aches for all the parents who are missing the pieces to the puzzle and are struggling through parenthood, trying to make their baby fit into someone else's mold.

The baby stage is short, but the days are long. I hope this book has given you confidence and the tools to *thrive*, not just survive.

Appendix

Recommended Routines

2 - 6 weeks
RECOMMENDED ROUTINE

7:00AM — Anchor Feed: Always start within 30 minutes of "scheduled" time.

Wake time: Keep wake window to 60 minutes or less.

8:00AM — 1st Nap: 90-120 minutes (hopefully)

10:00AM — 2nd Feed: Start as soon as baby wakes up. Scheduled time is not important here.

Wake time: Keep wake window to 60 minutes or less.

11:00AM — 2nd Nap: Duration doesn't matter.

12:30PM — 3rd Feed: Start as soon as baby wakes up.

Wake time: Keep wake window to 60 minutes or less.

1:30PM — 3rd Nap: At least 60 minutes (hopefully). Don't wake baby unless over 180 minutes.

3:30PM — 4th Feed: Start as soon as baby wakes up.

Wake time: Keep wake window to 45-60 minutes. Be mindful of stimulation.

4:30PM — 4th Nap: Duration doesn't matter.

5:30PM — 5th Feed: Start as soon as baby wakes up.

Wake time: Keep wake window to 60 minutes or less.

6:30PM — 5th Nap: Duration doesn't matter.

BEDTIME ROUTINE — (Maximum 10 minutes) Wake baby if still asleep at 8:00PM. This is the ONLY time you don't follow the feed, wake, sleep cycle.

BETWEEN 7PM-8PM — 6th Feed: Start right after bedtime routine.

BEDTIME — Follow nighttime feeding and sleep recommendations for feeds until the morning Anchor Feed.

BETWEEN 10PM-12AM — 7th Feed: Let baby wake up for this feed. Don't wake baby.

BETWEEN 1AM-3AM — 8th Feed: Let baby wake up for this feed. Don't wake baby.

BETWEEN 3-4AM — 9th Feed: Baby might possibly wake up for this feed. Don't wake baby.

NIGHTTIME WAKINGS

If baby wakes up before the 1st morning feeding (Anchor Feed), follow the guidelines for feeding and putting baby back to sleep.

Example: Anchor Feed is at 6:30. Baby wakes up at 5:00. Feed baby and follow nighttime rules (put baby back to sleep after feeding).

Wake baby within 30 minutes of Anchor Feed (by 7:00 AM in this example) even though she just ate at 5:00.

The Anchor Feed is the foundation for your daily routine. It may be the MOST important "rule" to follow!

You *can* do this. *Hillary*

Baby Settler™

6 weeks - 3 months
RECOMMENDED ROUTINE

7:00AM — Anchor Feed: Always start within 30 minutes of "scheduled" time.

Wake time: Keep wake window to 90 minutes or less.

8:00AM — 1st Nap: 90-120 minutes (hopefully)

10:00AM — 2nd Feed: Start as soon as baby wakes up.

Wake time: Keep wake window to 90 minutes or less.

11:00AM — 2nd Nap: Duration doesn't matter. (Usually 30-45 minutes)

12:30PM — 3rd Feed: Start as soon as baby wakes up.

Wake time: Keep wake window to 60 minutes or less.

1:30PM — 3rd Nap: At least 60 minutes (hopefully). Don't wake baby unless over 180 minutes.

3:30PM — 4th Feed: Start as soon as baby wakes up.

Wake time: Keep wake window to 45-60 minutes. Be mindful of stimulation.

4:30PM — 4th Nap: Duration doesn't matter. (Usually 30-45 minutes)

5:30PM — 5th Feed: Start as soon as baby wakes up.

Wake time: Keep wake window to 60 minutes or less.

6:30PM — 5th Nap: Duration doesn't matter. (Usually 30-45 minutes)

BEDTIME ROUTINE — (Maximum 10 minutes) Wake baby if still asleep at 8:00PM. This is the ONLY time you don't follow the feed, wake, sleep cycle.

BETWEEN 7PM-8PM — 6th Feed: Start right after bedtime routine.

BEDTIME — Follow nighttime feedings and sleep recommendations for all feeds until the morning Anchor Feed.

BETWEEN 11PM-12AM — 7th Feed: Let baby wake up for this feed. Don't wake baby.

BETWEEN 2-4AM — 8th Feed: Baby might possibly wake up for this feed. Don't wake baby.

NIGHTTIME WAKINGS

If baby wakes up before the 1st morning feeding (Anchor Feed), follow the guidelines for feeding and putting baby back to sleep.

Example: Anchor Feed is at 6:30. Baby wakes up at 5:00. Feed baby and follow nighttime rules (put baby back to sleep after feeding).

Wake baby within 30 minutes of Anchor Feed (by 7:00 AM in this example) even though she just ate at 5:00.

The Anchor Feed is the foundation for your daily routine. It may be the MOST important "rule" to follow!

You *can* do this. *Hillary*

Baby Settler™

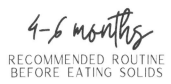

4-6 months

RECOMMENDED ROUTINE
BEFORE EATING SOLIDS

7:00AM — Anchor Feed: Always start within 30 minutes of "scheduled" time.

Wake time: Keep wake window to 90 minutes or less.

8:00AM — 1st Nap: 90-120 minutes (hopefully)

10:00AM — 2nd Feed: Start as soon as baby wakes up.

Wake time: Keep wake window to 2.5-3 hours or less.

12:00PM — 3rd Feed.

12:30PM — 2nd Nap: At least 90 minutes (hopefully). Don't wake baby unless over 180 minutes.

3:00PM — 4th Feed: Start as soon as baby wakes up.

Wake time: Be mindful of stimulation. Keep wake window to 2.5-3 hour max.

SHORT NAP — Possible short nap (30-45 minutes)

5:00PM — 5th Feed.

Wake time: Keep wake window to 90 minutes or less.

SHORT NAP — Possible short nap if baby did not nap after the 3:00 PM feed.

BEDTIME ROUTINE — Wake your baby if still asleep at 7:00 PM.

7:00PM — 6th Feed: Start right after bedtime routine.

BEDTIME — Follow nighttime feeding and sleep recommendations for all feeds until the morning Anchor Feed.

NIGHTTIME WAKINGS

If baby wakes up before the 1st morning feeding (Anchor Feed), follow the guidelines for feeding and putting baby back to sleep.

Example: Anchor Feed is at 6:30. Baby wakes up at 5:00. Feed baby and follow nighttime rules (put baby back to sleep after feeding).

Wake baby within 30 minutes of Anchor Feed (by 7:00 AM in this example) even though she just ate at 5:00.

The Anchor Feed is the foundation for your daily routine. It may be the MOST important "rule" to follow!

You *can* do this. Hilary

Baby Settler™

7-12 months

RECOMMENDED ROUTINE
ONCE EATING SOLIDS

7:00AM Anchor Feed: Offer complementary solids within 30 minutes of breast milk or formula feeding.

Wake time: Keep wake window to 60 minutes or less.

8:00AM Morning Nap: This nap will gradually get shorter in duration as baby approaches 10-12 months.

10:00AM 2nd Feed: Start as soon as baby wakes up.

Wake time: Keep wake window to 2.5-3 hours or less.

12:00PM 3rd Feed: You may offer complementary solids after breast milk or formula feeding.

12:45PM Midday Nap: 60 minutes to 3 hours

3:30PM 4th Feed: Start as soon as baby wakes up.

4-5PM You may offer complementary solids. Don't offer solids after 5:30 PM because baby won't take a full breast milk or formula feeding if he fills up on solids.

Wake time: Keep wake window to 3.5 hours or less. (Put baby to bed for the night 30 minutes early if she wakes from her midday nap early.)

6:15PM Bedtime Routine

6:30PM 5th Feed

7:00PM Bedtime

NIGHTTIME WAKINGS

If baby wakes up before the 1st morning feeding (Anchor Feed), review the video on Sleep Challenges in my *Babies* course.

You *can* do this. Hillary

Recommended Routines

Baby Settler™

12-18 months

RECOMMENDED ROUTINE
TO START ONCE NO LONGER
BREAST/BOTTLE FEEDING

7:00AM Breakfast

Wake time: Keep wake window to 60 minutes.

8:30AM Morning Nap: Most babies will continue this AM nap until about 15 months.

9:30AM Morning Snack

Wake time.

11:30AM Lunch

12:30PM Midday Nap: 60 minutes to 3 hours

3:00PM Afternoon snack

Wake time.

BETWEEN
5-6PM Dinner

6:30PM Bedtime Routine

7:00PM Bedtime

You *can* do this. *Hillary*

If you're looking for more information about birth, breastfeeding, and strategies for establishing daytime naps, extending nighttime sleep, or weaning nighttime feedings, the following online video courses are for you:

Birth Made Simple

Birth doesn't have to be intimidating or overwhelming.
(For parents who want to be prepared for childbirth.)

Breastfeeding Made Simple

Confidently make decisions and troubleshoot problems when breastfeeding your child.
(For breastfeeding mamas from birth to weaning.)

Babies Made Simple

Understand how feeding affects sleep and sleep affects feeding.
(Support for parents from birth through toddlerhood.)

"The information is informative but easy to understand and actually put to use. Understanding the "why" has been helpful in navigating our newborn's needs and not feeling like helpless new parents! The Babies Made Simple manual has been a great reference as our baby grows and we are able to quickly reference information or review different stages/needs as our baby's needs change. After taking these courses we felt empowered as parents and have been enjoying the newborn stage instead of stressed!" - Ashley

How to access this valuable information:

1. Sign up for the course at babysettler.com
2. Watch the videos you need, *when you need them* with access for 18 months.
3. During this season, *thrive*—don't just survive!